DOPEFIEND

Special Praise for *Dopefiend: A Father's Journey from Addiction to Redemption*

"In this brilliant memoir, Tim Elhajj illuminates what the long, hard road looks like for those of us who are in recovery or those of us who love someone in recovery. The daily effort, the scores of setbacks weathered, and small triumphs hard-earned that, in time, move us into a deep, intimate, authentic relationship to ourselves, to others, and to the world—one that we thought we'd never have; one that might not be what another might choose but that is what we require. I will keep this book near; I will give it to friends; I will cherish it always."

Louise DeSalvo
Author of Writing as a Way of Healing

*   *   *

"Tim Elhajj tells the story of his tenuous relationship with his son and his recovery from the heroin addiction he acquired during his childhood in a Pennsylvania steel town. While *Dopefiend* follows the twelve steps of a recovery program, these steps serve as the frame that hold together a sequence of masterly told vignettes. In one heartrending incident, Elhajj stands in line during a dismal Christmas to receive an already wrapped and donated toy for his son. Elhajj doesn't know his son's address. Sentiment is such a dangerous ground for most writers since it easily falls into sappiness; yet, Elhajj instinctively finds the right balance in telling his often gut-wrenching tale. *Dopefiend* should be put on the same shelf as William Burroughs's *Junkie* and Nick Flynn's *Another Bullshit Night in Suck City*."

Matt Briggs
Author of *The Remains of River Names* and *Shoot the Buffalo*

*   *   *

"This is an extremely moving and powerful memoir. Elhajj doesn't linger on the ugliness of addiction itself, but focuses on the solution and the hard road that as addicts and alcoholics we must all travel if we choose to turn our lives around. Elhajj is a fine writer and brave soul with a tremendous heart. His story is one of staggering loss and seemingly insurmountable struggles, but in the end he leaves us victorious, with the greatest message of all—one of hope and redemption."

James Brown
Author of *This River* and *The Los Angeles Diaries*

"I recommend Tim Elhajj's *Dopefiend* to anyone interested in chemical dependency and recovery from it. The book's subtitle, *A Father's Journey from Addiction to Redemption*, more accurately sums up its content. Like Franz Wright or Mary Karr, Elhajj lets the vivid details contained in his punchy prose make his points for him, without editorializing or preaching. The lean story that results gets right to the point: it's possible for an addict to change, with time and grace, from an inept and disconnected father to exactly the kind of example and confidante a son needs when the son has become an adult."

Fr. Jim Harbaugh, SJ
Author of *A 12-Step Approach to the Spiritual Exercises of St. Ignatius*

*   *   *

"This is a *real* book, about a person, who becomes a *real* person. The biggest mistake any of us can make in life is to make the outside world real and the inside one not. The author made this mistake. For too many years he believed the delusions his drug world provided him and never came close to discovering his true nature. Confusing pleasure for happiness he nearly destroyed himself. You don't have to be doing drugs to miss life. You can search for happiness in a million ways and not find it. As the author teaches us, it's what we stop doing that transforms our life. If you have ever wondered what goes on in that cocoon where the caterpillar turns into a butterfly, read this book."

Robert Smith, LCSW
Addiction Specialist and Interventionist

*   *   *

"I love this book! From the first page, I was swept up into the story and the narrator's progress from a Lower East Side homeless shelter to rehab and beyond. Most stories of addiction focus on the addiction side of the story and say little about what the actual work of recovery looks like. *Dopefiend* is a riveting portrayal of the recovery side of the equation. Both funny and poignant, this book belongs on the shelf beside the very best of recovery memoirs, such as Knapp's *Drinking: A Love Story* and Karr's *Lit*."

Theo Pauline Nestor
Author of *How to Sleep Alone in a King-Size Bed*

DOPEFIEND

A FATHER'S

JOURNEY FROM

ADDICTION TO

REDEMPTION

TIM ELHAJJ

To Jay!

Keep Coming

Back

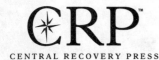

CENTRAL RECOVERY PRESS

CENTRAL RECOVERY PRESS

Central Recovery Press (CRP) is committed to publishing exceptional materials addressing addiction treatment, recovery, and behavioral health care, including original and quality books, audio/visual communications, and web-based new media. Through a diverse selection of titles, we seek to contribute a broad range of unique resources for professionals, recovering individuals and their families, and the general public.

For more information, visit www.centralrecoverypress.com.

Central Recovery Press, Las Vegas, NV 89129
©2011 by Tim Elhajj

ISBN 10: 1-936290-63-4
ISBN 13: 978-1-936290-63-5

17 16 15 14 13 12 11   1 2 3 4 5

Publisher: Central Recovery Press
              3321 N Buffalo Drive
              Las Vegas, NV 89129

Publisher's Note: This is a memoir; a work based on fact recorded to the best of the author's memory. CRP books represent the experiences and opinions of their authors only. Every effort has been made to ensure that events, institutions, and statistics presented in our books as facts are accurate and up-to-date. The opinions expressed are those of the authors only. To protect their privacy, the names of some of the people and institutions in this book have been changed.

The chapter "Honesty" first appeared in *Brevity* as "Jimi Don't Play Here No More." Author's photo by Kennedy Elhajj. Copyright ©2009. Used by permission.

Excerpt from *This Boy's Life*, copyright ©1989 by Tobias Wolff. Used by permission of Grove/Atlantic, Inc.

Cover design and interior by Sara Streifel, Think Creative Design

For
Timothy, Aaron, Kennedy,
Jasmine, and Jade

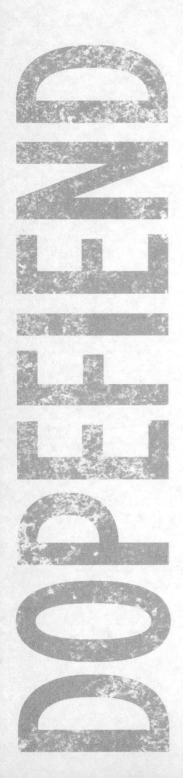

TABLE OF CONTENTS

ACKNOWLEDGMENTS

I'd like to thank Holly Huckeba for her insightful comments and many close readings of this book. In the final days of pulling the manuscript through revision, I thought I was losing my mind. Each time that happened, Holly helped me find it again. What a great friend. I'd also like to thank Gary Presley, Grace Skibicki, Diane Diekman, Kathleen Purcell and the many other participants of the nonfiction group at The Internet Writing Workshop for their support, advice, and encouragement. This is a much better book as a result of their help.

After I got out of rehab this last time, I tried to work the Twelve Steps perfectly. I struggled with the idea of progress, not perfection. A friend of mine took me aside and said, "Each day you stay away from drugs and alcohol, you work one or more of the steps whether you know it or not." What a relief. I've tried to make progress with the steps this same way for more than twenty years now. But some habits die hard, and while writing this book, I again tried to be perfect—getting each detail completely accurate. At one point, my son pointed out that one of the vehicles I had remembered as a truck was actually a compact car. In the spirit of progress, not perfection, I am standing by my own fuzzy memory and allowing some of these discrepancies to stand. For, as Tobias Wolff pointed out in *This Boy's Life*, "memory has its own story to tell."

AUTHOR'S NOTE

I want to thank my publisher, CRP, for giving me the opportunity to write about my recovery. CRP bought this manuscript on proposal, which means that the book hadn't been completed when it was purchased. I think it's safe to say that we were all surprised with what I eventually produced. I was delighted by how well it turned out. CRP, meanwhile, seemed a little taken aback with some of my experiences and even the way in which I told about them. You'll find mostly deceit in the chapter titled "Honesty." A zombie appears in the chapter titled "Faith." And let's not even get into what happens in the "Integrity" chapter. We traded emails. We had phone calls. I wasn't sure what would happen. Finally, Nancy Schenck, the Executive Editor at CRP, told me she would support my vision for this book. I am so grateful for the faith that she has placed in me and in my story.

I am the first to admit that my recovery has not followed the typical path you hear about in most meetings. I am not one for moralizing, nor am I eager to play the role of provocateur. However, I do feel strongly that our stories are the most powerful tools we own. To shape our stories to fit some preconceived mold is unfair to people new to recovery, who may be struggling to understand what changes need to be wrought in their own lives and who may be interested in reading an accurate expression of another's experience.

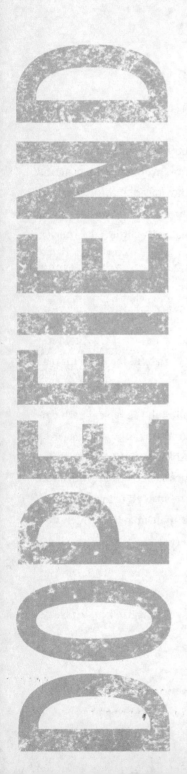

PROLOGUE

More than twenty years ago, I moved to New York City with less than twenty dollars in my pocket to kick a heroin habit. I was leaving behind my beautiful three-year-old boy, who had his mother's straw-colored hair and clear blue eyes, exactly the opposite of my own dark hair and eyes. I searched for some recognizable piece of myself in his chipper, smiling face but didn't see much.

I was twenty-six and leaving Steelton, the small town in south-central Pennsylvania where I had grown up amid high school football games, Bethlehem Steel, and the shallow waters of the Susquehanna River. Nine years earlier I had first shot up heroin here. No drug I tried in high school had ever made me feel the way heroin did. After finishing with the military, I returned home, eager to resume using this drug. My friends and I mocked the older heroin addicts we knew, many of whom still lived in their mother's houses, slept in their childhood beds, and rarely dated or did anything other than chase heroin. Unlike those guys, I soon married a girl a few years younger than myself. My addiction seemed to stir some strange mix of benevolence and fascination in her. She would set little abstinence tasks for me to perform, and these I cheerfully subverted or undermined. I felt confident that once I found a comfortable groove, I would throw off my expensive habit.

When my wife got pregnant, I knew I ought to stop. But as she gave birth in the hospital, I raced from the waiting room to purchase Dilaudid, a fancy name for pharmaceutical heroin. In our bedroom, I would stare at my infant son's tiny fingers and delicate nails, so pink and magnificent, and realize I hadn't a clue how to be a good father. Soon my wife took him and left.

I rallied to win them back. My mother suggested a drug treatment program with her Charismatic Christian Church. But I ended up as unenthusiastic for religion as my son's mother was for my efforts in treatment. Soon I began hanging out with the older addicts I used to mock and getting into real trouble with the Steelton police.

I ended up in drug treatment again, this time at a secular facility. Attending my first recovery meeting, I found many of my friends were starting off their own recovery this way. In the course of a "reconciliation" effected by the rehab facility, my wife made it clear we were through. Whatever spark she once carried for me had long since flickered out.

Moving on, I tried to figure out how to be a good parent, but I still hadn't even figured out how to remain abstinent. During the short bursts of recovery I did manage, I'd show up with presents or for some daddy time.

Even as a toddler, my son made his interest in athletics clear: He would clamor to watch any sport with a ball on TV, even golf. As a boy, I'd always done terribly in sports. During my childhood, I'd watched with growing alarm, and then envy, as my older brothers developed into excellent athletes. So why, I wondered, had God made me the father of this sturdy, sports-minded boy? With each relapse, I grew more cynical. Soon all my friends were celebrating their first years in recovery, and I was still mired in addiction.

During this time, there was a guy I knew who had been a heroin addict himself but had been in recovery for about five years: Buster B. At the time, it seemed unimaginable to me that anyone who had once used heroin could go so long without the drug. Buster was stocky with an open, friendly face. He had a receding hairline and wore his blond hair in a carefully greased crew cut, a slick curb of clipped hair rising and falling across his forehead like a McDonald's sign. To ward off the coming winter, he wore a long pea coat. Buster liked to wear black Wayfarer sunglasses, a host of gold rings on his fingers, and thick ropes of gold chain around his neck. He had a beautiful girlfriend, a busty redhead who smoked long brown cigarettes. Buster always drove a new Ford sedan with dealer plates attached by magnets to the trunk. When dopefiends get into recovery, they invariably seem to do one of two things to make a living: car sales or drug and alcohol counseling. Buster worked at the big Ford dealership on Paxton and Cameron Streets, but he liked to show up to the recovery meetings and do a little impromptu counseling on the side. We envied his jewelry, his shiny sedan, his pneumatic girlfriend. But it was his recovery time that held us in awe. Milling about during a smoke break at the meeting, we sipped coffee from Styrofoam cups and listened to whatever Buster had to say.

"There are only two things you need to do to stay in recovery," Buster said.

We all raised our eyebrows. We'd heard in meetings that there were at least twelve things, even if we couldn't articulate exactly what those things were. Yet here was Buster talking about doing only two. Seemed like a bargain. We all shuffled in a little bit closer.

"First," Buster said. "Don't get high."

This was an obvious first step, and a little chuckle rose up from the seven or eight of us standing there. If you're not an addict, it may seem like this solves the entire problem. It does not. The list of things that can impose a moratorium on street drug use is endless. Someone gets pinched somewhere along the distribution chain and suddenly there are no drugs available. You have to stop. Or one day you might not be able to get your money together. And, you can always get busted yourself. Not getting high is as much a part of getting high as being able to poke a vein or get your money together. And let's not forget about the legal highs like sex, gambling, and alcohol. The trick isn't to stop using, but to remain abstinent for the long haul.

"Second," Buster said.

And here he paused for effect and held up two fingers. This was the money step: the crucial information we needed to stay in recovery. The signet ring on Buster's stubby pinky glittered in the afternoon sun. I didn't want to seem too eager, but I couldn't help but feel that I was about to hear something momentous. I leaned in a little closer.

Buster had a little half-smile on his lips as he sipped his coffee and adjusted his coat.

"Boys," he said. He glanced to his left and then to the right. When he was sure he had our undivided attention, he said, "Change your whole fucking life around."

He laughed heartily at his own little joke and stroked his tummy. The rest of us stood there in silence. Buster crushed out his cigarette and grinned. "Come on," he said, walking past us. "Let's get back to the meeting."

Fucking Buster B.

He was just toying with us then, but I have come to realize that Buster B's little joke wasn't all that far from the truth. To make the most of recovery, I would have to change just about every aspect of my life: I would need a spiritual, emotional, and intellectual makeover of the most sweeping kind.

Of course, I didn't understand any of this back then. None of us did.

We all groaned and smirked and scowled. Someone shook his head. Another person laughed good-naturedly and mumbled, "Cocksucker." We were a forlorn little group of barely recovering addicts, who thought we had stumbled upon a good deal. Instead we had the same old dusty twelve "To Dos" we started with.

The only way to get where I wanted to go, it seemed, was to do all twelve.

And in New York, this is exactly what I did. It was a good thing, too. As it turned out, my son grew from a beautiful blond boy to a strapping hulk of a young man. Today, he towers over me, his eyes still blue, his hair still clipped short. Over the years, he has looked skeptically at my long locks, my affinity for faded black jeans and combat boots, and my deep disinterest in athleticism of any kind. The one thing we have in common is a penchant for self-destruction: This is the most recognizable piece of me that I have found in him. The only way I could hope to offer him much as a parent was to first find my own way through the maze of addiction to recovery.

Here, then, is my story in twelve chapters: a chapter for each step, a step for each chapter.

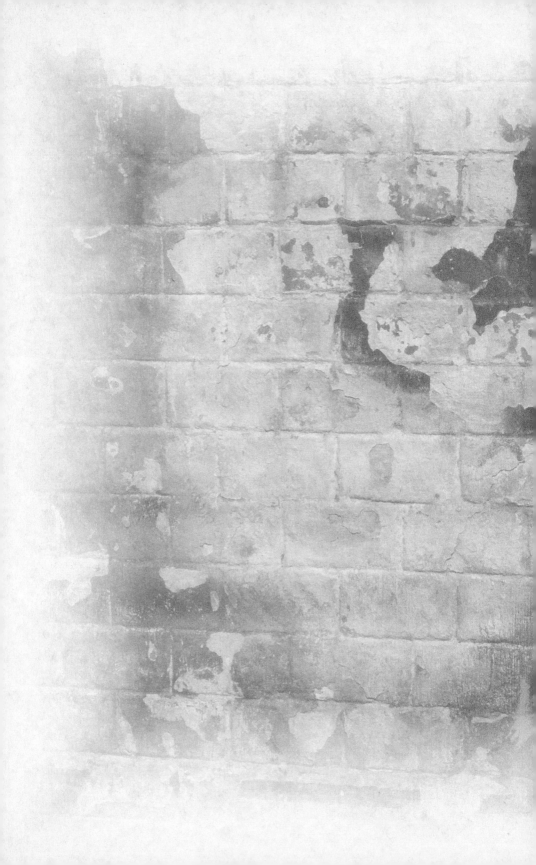

CHAPTER 1

HONESTY

After getting booted from high school three times, I joined the military. Three years into my enlistment, the Navy cut me loose. I moved back to Pennsylvania and got married, but soon after our first child was born, my wife split, taking our baby boy with her.

I was a twenty-four-year-old cyclone of poor decisions.

In time, I landed in county jail. At least nobody gets thrown out of jail. Drug treatment followed, but even that didn't work: I went to recovery meetings high. One night a woman named Wendy R pulled me aside and hissed: "You are going to die!"

I told her the obvious, "We're all going to die, Wendy."

Another court date loomed. I was too soft for more jail. In a bid for leniency from the judge, I decided to enter drug treatment again. Although the rehabs in Pennsylvania refused to take me back, they suggested a facility up in the Bronx.

I assessed my situation. New York City seemed like a long shot, another poor decision, in a lifetime of poor decisions. But it seemed as if it'd be the only shot I'd have.

I took the Greyhound to Times Square, arriving with the chilly December daylight. Steam billowed from grates, cars packed the streets, and long morning shadows fell like knives.

I made my way to a drug bazaar in Alphabet City. My last fix, my last twenty dollars. I walked to 99th and Amsterdam for an intake appointment, and what would be my last stop before the Bronx. Around 3:00 p.m., a social worker named Roberto started my paperwork. He had greasy hair and wore a button down shirt that appeared to have been created from a Puerto Rican flag. He asked when the last time I got high was. I was nervous and thought a joke might lighten the mood.

"What time is it now?" I asked.

"You got high today?" Roberto scowled. Instead of sending me to the Bronx, he told me to go back downtown to a homeless shelter.

"Get outta here," he said.

I balked. Why had I been truthful with Roberto? I needed treatment, not a homeless shelter. When he saw my distress, something in Roberto's manner softened, but he stayed firm about the shelter. I had to go.

I rode the train to the East Village. The shelter was on Saint Mark's Place. About a dozen homeless people wandered about in a damp and cavernous room with soaring black walls, large hand-painted hippie flowers, and purple peace signs.

"What is this place?" I asked.

"The Electric Circus," said a slight Latino with glassy eyes. "A night club from the 60s. Hendrix played here." A disco ball hung from the ceiling and fold-out cots were clustered in twos and threes on the dance floor. Looking around, I thought, one thing's for sure: Jimi don't play here no more.

Food was scarce. Weekdays, everyone would sit on the front steps to ask passers-by for change. I couldn't bring myself to beg. One morning, I went to the corner deli and slipped two ice cream sandwiches into my jacket. I could see little tornados of trash and fallen leaves swirling up the street.

"You," a tousle-headed man from behind the counter said. "Put those back."

I feigned innocence, but his dark eyes shone fiercely. "The ice cream in your jacket," he said. "Put it back."

I did as he asked and headed for the door.

"You hungry?" he asked. Without waiting for an answer, he sailed an oven-soft roll over the counter toward me. His kindness made my face burn with shame.

Weekends at the shelter, they held dances to raise funds. These lasted until 3:00 or 4:00 a.m., and you couldn't set up your cot until they were over. I just wanted to hide from all the handsome people, so I went to the basement, which everyone called the Dom. I was told the Dom had been Andy Warhol's, "Exploding Plastic Inevitable," as if this explained everything. Now the Dom was home to round-the-clock recovery meetings.

At one meeting, the chairperson started reading a passage from the program literature, then abruptly, without missing a word, he got up and headed to the back of the room, where an old homeless man had fallen asleep holding a lit cigar, setting his overcoat ablaze. The chairperson only stopped reading long enough to swat the flames out.

Good God, I thought.

In Pennsylvania, I had boosted a pair of Nikes: hi-top leather, white-on-white, my favorite kind of sneaker. I considered swapping these to another homeless guy who might have had some dope. As I was trying to decide what to do, the person in charge at the shelter, a beautiful Puerto Rican woman with an ugly scar that ran from the left side of her mouth all the way to her ear (this meant she had snitched), asked everyone to help decorate a pathetic little plastic tree someone had rescued from the trash—our Christmas tree.

There were no ornaments or lights: just newspaper folded into origami and some macaroni noodles threaded with string.

I decided it was beneath me.

Sitting in the corner, I cupped my hands to light a cigarette. I could hear the wind begin to rise and swirl around me. If everything worked out exactly the way I wanted—best case scenario—I would be high for a few hours, and then. . .

I would be barefoot.

In the city.

In December.

I decided I had better start decorating that ugly little tree.

CHAPTER 2

HOPE

Two weeks after arriving in New York City, I watched a dark blue van with side windows pull to the curb and idle in front of the homeless shelter. The woman on duty said I should climb in. I was going to the Bronx for treatment.

I piled into the middle seat of a van fully loaded with people: all of them sullen, quiet, and black. We wound through early afternoon traffic. Wipers slapped cold sleet from the windshield. I watched the gaily decorated downtown cityscape grow more desolate: soon we were passing lone tenement buildings, defiant hulks squatting in the middle of trash-strewn lots. We drove past the ornate splendor of Yankee Stadium and the Grand Concourse, a testament to better times. Soon the streets twisted and looped, making me feel as if I were entering a great labyrinth.

Nestled on the side of a hill, the Rockford facility was an enormous building, its steep walls rising up from the street below like the ramparts of some ancient castle. I could hear traffic on the Cross Bronx Expressway and trains rumbling past on the elevated Number Four line. Getting out of the van, I discreetly stretched. I was grateful to be out of the shelter, but wary of my new surroundings, and didn't want to call undue attention to myself. Waving his thick hands, a large bald man with gold caps on his teeth climbed out from the front passenger seat and directed us inside. From the way he seemed to enjoy flashing both his grin and his authority over us, I assumed he was a counselor—though I came to learn he was a client, like me.

In the lobby, people carrying clipboards directed those of us who had come from the van to sit on a raggedy collection of castaway furniture. Everyone holding a clipboard was black. I wondered what I had gotten myself into. Several women, some with hair braided into thick ropes, all with dark and gleaming skin, lingered in one corner of the lobby, quietly murmuring to one another.

Gold Teeth curtly barked orders to his co-workers. To those of us who had just gotten off the van, he showed a benign indifference, walking through our midst like we were pigeons clustered around his feet in the park. But to his peers, those other clipboard-wielding men, he behaved menacingly, demanding answers, calling for paperwork, and looking generally displeased with everyone's performance. It occurred to me he might be showing off for the women. This insight surprised me. I felt no sexual attraction toward this raw gang of women. If anything, they frightened me. More than one had lumped-up purple razor scars running across the fleshy skin of her arm or back. Some had bruised, ashen faces. But most unsettling was their sturdy and silent indifference, as they stood with chins jutted out or fists curled into plump hips.

That night I lay in the bottom half of a bunk bed in an open dormitory. Someone flashed the overhead lights to signal they would soon be shut off. There were at least two dozen of us packed into the large second-floor room, which had bathroom facilities at one end. Bunk beds were pushed against all the walls and people mostly stood in the center aisle of the room, chatting or milling about as they got ready for bed. Outside I could hear the low hum of traffic from the expressway and the occasional siren wail from somewhere in the city.

Considering where I was, I felt generally pleased and optimistic. The room was crowded but warm, a huge step up from the damp shelter on Saint Mark's Place. I felt as if it would be okay to remove my street clothes before I went to bed, which I hadn't done since arriving in the city. Dinner had been a baked chicken leg and thigh, a plop of mashed potatoes, and diced carrots. Because I was new, those in charge let me get seconds. I had bagged the bulk of my clothes and dropped them in a great canvas cart, ready to be laundered. My court appearance in Pennsylvania was scheduled for late February, about ten weeks out. I had done all I could to ensure I wouldn't end up in jail, and now felt certain the worst of this adventure was behind me.

Just as the lights went out, I heard three or four dull, popping sounds from the street below.

There was a lull in the dormitory conversation, but nobody seemed concerned by this noise. I immediately got off the bed. Gunshots? But the popping noise seemed so innocent, not at all like the crack of gunfire on TV. In a hurry to look out the window, I had to make my way to the room's center aisle and double back between bunks.

Someone called out, "Where you going?"

"You hear that?" I asked. Arriving at the window, I found my view of the street blocked. I turned and headed across the room; somewhere there had to be an unobstructed view.

"Don't look out the window," that same voice said.

Ignoring this advice, I squeezed between two bunks on the other side of the room, much closer to where I imagined the sounds had come from. "I want to see," I said.

"You'll get shot."

The unseen speaker's tone was somehow both plaintive and blunt. It wasn't a command, more a simple statement of fact. I pulled up short. Nobody else had made a move to the windows. Coming back to the center aisle, I grinned at the person speaking to me.

"Good point," I said.

Mike introduced himself. He was the blackest black man I had ever seen. He wore a tight white T-shirt and folded his muscular arms across his chest. His skin was so black, shadow didn't seem to register on his face or arms, giving him an unsettling two-dimensional appearance, except for the cut of his strong chest, which showed in relief against the cotton of his shirt. Mike grinned, a toothy white smile. "If it was gunshots, you don't want to see."

"I didn't even think of that," I said. He had a magazine folded in three and tucked under his arm. He looked about twenty-two years old, which would make him five years younger than me. There were a few other young men standing nearby him.

"Where you from, Country?" Mike asked.

"Pennsylvania," I said. Feeling a little put off by the nickname, I added: "It's only four hours out of the city."

"Is Pennsylvania south?" he asked.

I nodded, amused by what I took for his lack of geographic awareness.

"Then that's the country," he said. All his friends laughed. "You from the country, Country." Mike grinned.

His smile lit up his face, emphasizing his boyish good looks. I found it hard to stay annoyed at him.

"What you got there," I asked, nodding to the magazine under his arm, just to change the subject.

"Porn," he said, tugging the magazine out and handing it to me.

"Oh..." My voice rose unintentionally. Pornographic magazines were most likely contraband. A small infraction to be sure, but I hadn't intended to break any rules. My job was to stay out of trouble until after my court date. With all the guys looking at me, I felt as if it would have been rude to refuse the magazine, so I took it and held it in front of me. "Is having porn against the rules?" I asked.

"Yup," Mike said. There was an awkward silence. "You going to tell?" He cocked his head and I could hear mild disbelief.

"No, no, no," I said. Breaking the rules was bad, but being labeled a snitch was certainly much worse. "I just wondered," I said.

"A'ight." Mike looked at me evenly. "Go take care of that thing," he nodded toward the bathroom. "Then bring me back my magazine."

"Oh, right," I laughed nervously.

I felt a sudden and jarring shock at the way the conversation had turned. The small group that had formed around us scrutinized me. "Right," I repeated.

Feeling self-conscious, I wasn't sure how to gracefully exit the little group. I started to walk backwards toward the bathroom, waving the magazine around in front of me, like some circus buffoon. I tripped over something in the aisle and then laughed nervously again at my own awkwardness.

Mike and each of his friends looked at one another and shook their heads. Someone clucked his teeth. I felt grateful for the darkness in the room, for I could feel my face getting hot.

* * *

One week into treatment, I was making my way back to the dormitory after Evening Focus. Focus meetings were held twice daily, morning and evening, in a large auditorium on the first floor. One of the counselors, a short man named Angel, was standing in the hallway, urging anyone who was a parent to go to the north wing of the first floor where the administrative offices were. The hallways on the first floor were always packed after focus meetings and meals, but especially during the workday morning and evening rush.

"You got a kid." Angel said to me. "Over there," he pointed. It wasn't a question and he didn't wait for an answer. He gave my shoulder a little shove.

Jostling my way through the crowd, I made my way to the north wing and found a line of people that stretched the length of the building. I went to the end of the line and stood, wondering why I was there.

I asked the person in front of me, but he had no idea. Five minutes later the line had not budged, but another person or two had come to stand behind me. None of us understood why we were here. Growing impatient, I made my way to the front of the line.

As I asked further up, someone said, "Toys."

Craning my neck, I could see a counselor listlessly sitting in an office with a great pile of packages behind him. Inside the office, a person from the line stood rubbing his chin as he surveyed the stack of packages.

"Donations," I heard someone else say.

Donated toys. We were standing in line to select a donated Christmas toy for our kids. I could feel something terrible rising in my chest. As I walked back to my place at the end of the line, I felt myself growing agitated and irritable.

I wasn't sure where my son lived. It had been months since I'd seen him. He would be four years old the month after Christmas. I knew his mother had recently moved, from Shamokin back to Steelton, but I wasn't sure if she was staying with her mother now, or on her own. Last I heard she was seeing Jack Driscoll, who owned a house across the street from my mother's house.

Standing in line, I began to feel distressed. I sighed heavily and ran my fingers through my hair. I wasn't particularly concerned with getting a toy, but I complained aloud about the length of the line and fidgeted.

"This is so stupid," I said to no one in particular.

"You too good for our toys?" Rick, a lanky counselor with a bald head, had come out of one of the nearby offices. His presence surprised me; his sharp tone put me on guard. I hadn't meant to draw attention to myself.

"No," I stammered. "No. . ."

"What's up?" he asked.

"I just feel. . ." I had to think for a minute.

Groping for the right word, I finally said: "Bad." I winced at my inability to convey what I was feeling. Suddenly I felt my eyes well with tears. The intensity and speed of my emotions shocked me. "Really bad," I added.

He looked me directly in the eye. He didn't smile, but something in his manner softened. "You feel bad because you're in treatment and have to get your kid a donated toy for Christmas," he said.

I shrugged. "I don't even know where to send it," I admitted.

With these words, my irritability disappeared and despair took its place. I felt limp and useless, like a wet towel on a clothesline in the middle of a downpour.

* * *

Immediately after the holiday lull, Rockford went into an uproar. The entire community filed into the auditorium for Morning Focus, a meeting typically only attended by the facility's newest members. Vans had been halted, the laundry shuttered, and the administrative wing locked down. The kitchen remained open for breakfast, but only a skeleton crew remained to clean up and prepare a simple lunch. Something was going on.

As the auditorium filled, I took a seat in the right wing, close to the stage. There were at least five hundred people seated and still more passing through the double doors. The quiet roar of confusion filled the great space. I could hear senior members complain about the vans being stopped: They were missing work, trade programs, or appointments at clinics or social service offices. The gang of women I had seen in the lobby on my first day was led into the great hall in a group. A wiry woman, evidently in authority, fluttered about them, chirping directions in a Hispanic accent and watching carefully as they made their way toward the rows of seats reserved for them. A hush seemed to fall across the crowd in the vicinity of the women as they passed, as if the wiry woman's scrutiny alone were enough to suppress noise.

A group of counselors took the stage. Juan, a short Latino, pleaded for quiet over the microphone. Ramon, stocky and balding, used his hands like a traffic cop. But the noise kept rising. Then, Terrance Tyson, a counselor from East New York, one of the toughest, most desperate crack-torn neighborhoods in all of Brooklyn, took the microphone from Juan and barked, "Shut the fuck up!"

The sudden silence was followed almost immediately by a ripple of laughter. All of the counselors reacted quickly to the laughter, swearing and berating the entire community until there was utter stillness. This was meant to be a somber occasion.

Taking the stage next was James, the director of the program, an athletic-looking man whose youthful countenance was belied by his gray temples. As the director paced, the auditorium grew tense. He spoke in a low tone that felt menacing. Gold Teeth and two of his peers were led onstage. The three of them stood, stoop-shouldered, staring at their shoes, like sinners in church. Of all the client jobs, these men's had been the highest positions of authority. I was shocked to see them singled out like this.

James went on about clients breaking the rules. He was coy about specifics. It became clear he wanted the specifics from us. Looking across the seats, I saw mostly teenagers and young men, crackheads from some of the worst neighborhoods in New York City.

Good luck, I thought.

Next James called a young man in baggy jeans and hooded jacket on stage. This boy had been remanded to treatment by the courts with a significant amount of jail time hanging in the balance. He seemed oddly pleased by this fact, as if it lent him a stature he might not otherwise have been able to attain. In group, he liked to refer to himself—proudly and with no irony—as a predicate felon. "Yo, I'm a predicate felon."

I found him arrogant and disagreeable but could see the fear in his eyes and felt bad for him now. He was shaking his head, denying any wrongdoing.

"Get your shit," James told him, "and get the fuck out."

"What that mean?" Predicate Felon's voice filled with emotion. "I don't understand."

"You don't understand?" James snorted. "Well, okay. Let's break it down. 'Get your shit' *mean*, go upstairs and get your stuff." James paused. Speaking directly into the microphone, he said: "'Get the fuck out,' *mean* 'Get the fuck out.'"

His amplified voice echoed from the walls.

Predicate Felon's shoulders slumped.

Turning his attention from the boy, James addressed the crowd. He wanted us to tell on ourselves, tell on our friends, and tell on one another. James wanted this information now.

For the rest of the day a parade of counselors appeared on stage, alone or sometimes in pairs. They alternated between cursing and berating us, or making impassioned pleas for us to discuss any rule infractions we might know of. I didn't mind the cursing, but by the time evening came, the pleas were taking their toll. Something about the soothing promise of redemption and the measured cadence of the counselor's arguments put me on edge.

People were beginning to crack.

One by one they raised their hands, like churchgoers making an altar call, and were led out by counselors to the administrative wing. I saw Mike briefly at dinner, but we weren't allowed to talk.

Gold Teeth split, storming off the stage late evening on day two. Others slipped out during the night. A quiet desperation seemed to settle over everyone, even the counselors whose curses and taunts now rang softly in our ears. Sometimes they let us sit in the auditorium for hours in silence.

After dinner the third day, Ramon led me and half a dozen other new people to the administrative wing. Ramon started in on his plea for information. Halfway through his spiel, Ramon began pacing the hall in front of us as he spoke. He seemed exasperated. I decided I couldn't take it anymore. I would tell about the porn magazine.

I raised my hand.

"You fucking guys are all brand new—," Ramon said.

I waved my hand.

"You haven't been here long enough to know shit." He ran his hand over the shiny skin of his head.

Ramon looked at me with bloodshot eyes. He chuckled with a derisive snort. "Jesus fucking Christ."

I lowered my hand.

"What the fuck?" He hiked his pants. "What do you want?"

Tongue-tied, I shrugged my shoulders and said nothing. Rockford was a madhouse—of this much I was certain. In my desperation to avoid jail and get into treatment, I had signed on at an asylum.

* * *

Days after the lockdown ended, I piled into a van with Mike and a few others to go downtown to a public clinic for physicals and blood tests, a standard procedure for all new clients.

We drove into Manhattan and were dropped off in a public park nearby the clinic to wait for it to open. Homeless people wandered the park in the early morning light: some rooted through trash, while others pushed carts, or rested on sodden sheets of cardboard laid on the bare, wet ground.

"What's up with all these hobos?" I asked. "They're all over the place."

Mike cut his eyes at me and scowled.

"No seriously," I asked. "Why does New York have so many hobos?"

"Stop saying hobo, motherfucker," Mike said. He was sitting on the back of a park bench, with his feet on the seat. He blew into his cupped hands for warmth and then looked at me pointedly. "Wasn't you in the homeless shelter?"

"Yep," I grinned. "I was a hobo my damn self."

Mike snorted and shook his head.

"They ain't hobos, man. They homeless people," he said. He sounded irritated. He looked wistfully at the locked door of the clinic. "They got homeless people in Pennsylvania, too," he added. "They all over."

A pigeon fluttered down, landing on the concrete sidewalk. I watched it peck for crumbs as I shifted my weight from foot to foot. Hugging my crossed arms to my chest, I watched my breath turn to steam.

For a while, no one said anything. The pigeons cooed.

"If I got thrown out of the house," I said, almost in a whisper. "I just slept on the couch over at Bud's, or sometimes up at Mary and Frank's. . ."

* * *

In late February, I took the train back to Pennsylvania alone, to appear in court. Arriving in Harrisburg on Sunday afternoon, I phoned my mother-in-law from the train station. She listened as I asked to speak to her daughter, and then without saying a word to me, she cupped the receiver with her hand. I heard muffled voices and seconds later Maryanne answered.

"Can I see Joey?" I asked. "I'm only in town for the night."

She told me she was staying with Jack now, and that I was welcome to come and see Joey, but that there could be no trouble. She stressed the word trouble.

I took the bus to Jack's. The sky had gone dark purple, bringing the street lights up. The moon shone. To avoid walking past my mother's house, I climbed the concrete steps on Fourth and Swatara. Bethlehem Steel's dark stacks loomed even darker in silhouette against the night sky—straight and hard, like the cold iron bars of a prison cell. From Jack's front porch, I could see my mother's house and her car parked in the vacant lot up the street.

I wasn't welcome there.

At the door, Jack smiled and waved me inside. Joey came storming out of the dining room, screaming in delight. I had only enough time to drop my bag and make some hurried hellos, before he dragged me into the dining room to show me his birthday toys. Jack came into the dining room. He was about thirty-two, five years older than me, with a deep voice, working-man hands, and blonde hair in a crew cut.

Joey's blue eyes sparkled. The dining room floor was littered with toy cars and trucks. He sat across the room from Jack and me, and waved vaguely in our direction. "Dad! Dad! Hand me that car."

I held up a little blue '69 Camaro. "This?" I asked.

"No!" Joey happily shook his shorn head. "My other Dad." Jack rolled a Ford wagon over to Joey, who grinned ear-to-ear, and sent it roaring down the plastic track. With his light coloration, I noted ruefully that Joey looked more like Jack's son than he did mine.

Maryanne came down from upstairs, asked if I were hungry, and then darted into the kitchen. Jack wandered into the living room to watch TV. I followed Maryanne into the kitchen. She stood at the countertop, deftly assembling a sandwich. Thin, blonde, determined. Sandwich made, she turned from her task, shoved the plate into my hands and immediately headed for the other room.

"Wait, Mary—" I said. I was whispering and not even sure why.

"What?" Maryanne asked impatiently, her voice flat. She looked up at me with one eyebrow raised. There was an awkward pause, which I didn't know how to fill.

"He calls him Dad?" I asked.

"Tim," Maryanne said. "I do not want to hear the shit."

She tilted her head sweetly, and then left me standing in Jack's kitchen with a bologna sandwich and some potato chips.

I went into the dining room and raced cars with Joey. Later on, he showed me his room, with which he seemed delighted. Too soon, it was time for me to go. Maryanne asked if I were going across the street to visit my mother.

"I don't think so," I said. "No."

"You should go," Maryanne said. "She wants to see you."

"Doubtful," I mumbled.

"No. I called her," Maryanne said. "She definitely wants to see you."

"You called her?" My voice rose. Having someone else make the call for me hadn't even occurred to me, but knowing Maryanne had called seemed somehow unimaginable—Maryanne and my mom had never been close.

"What did she say?" I asked, alarmed.

Maryanne slowly enunciated: "She said . . . she wants . . . to see you."

Her consideration felt good, but her confidence that my mother wanted to see me left me feeling awkward, uncomfortable. At a loss for words, I hugged Joey, grabbed my bag, and made for the door.

"Thanks," I said.

Maryanne waved her hand, dismissing her kindness.

Joey howled with disappointment.

Across the street, I tapped on my mother's front door. After a few minutes, the curtain was pulled back. Mom; small, worn. A tight little knot of worry. Opening the door, she looked me up and down. Her hair was different now, short.

"Leave that there," she said, indicating my bag. "No one will mess with it."

I dropped the bag and followed her inside. One of my younger brothers was on the floor of the living room watching TV. Someone else was in the kitchen, but I couldn't tell who. I was about to sit on the couch, but Mom indicated a kitchen chair she had dragged into the middle of the living room.

I felt uncomfortable and started to talk. Yammer, really. I told her about the weather in New York, how big Joey was, the furniture in Jack's living room. Once I started, I didn't dare stop. As I went on, I realized Mom was clutching her purse to her chest. This astonished me. I had never seen her act with such undisguised caution. One time when I still lived here, I had overheard her tell my younger brother that she thought I might be Satan. Not that I was possessed, but that I was actually Satan. *"He goes through locked doors,"* she'd said, her voice desperate, edgy.

"Okay," Mom was saying, glancing at her watch. "You better go."

My throat was dry from talking. About fifteen minutes had passed. More than anything, I felt relieved it was over. On the front porch, she wished me luck and gave me a quick hug, which surprised me.

"Write," she said.

I was staying in a room over the Alva Restaurant, right next door to the train station, within walking distance of the court house. The kind of room prostitutes and their johns used by the hour. After my guilty plea was entered, I was duly remanded to treatment. I vaguely considered not going back to New York City, but the idea of staying near home gave me a bad feeling.

On the train ride back to Manhattan, I wondered about the unexpected visit with my mother. She'd asked me to write. Me. Write her.

I resolved I would.

*　*　*

Spring rolled in hot.

One afternoon at the rehab facility, I was sitting in the Vehicles Office with Aaron, one of the drivers. Aaron had a broad forehead, a quick wit, and thin brown hair that he wore pushed straight back. We had the morning shuttle route, which left at 7:00 a.m., and was usually done by noon, having us both back at the facility by 2:00 p.m. Vehicles was a cushy job.

Reading the *New York Times,* Aaron tipped his thick glasses up onto his nose. I sipped coffee from a paper cup. Another driver, Keith, poked his head into the office and shook the shaggy mop of blonde hair from his eyes. Keith tapped his fist to his chest, and then held up three fingers.

Looking up from his paper, Aaron grinned and made the same gesture.

"What's that?" I asked.

"*Wehicles,*" Aaron said, tipping his glasses higher on his nose. He held up three splayed fingers to make a W.

Keith grinned.

Creasing my brow, I shrugged. "Wehicles?"

Aaron looked surreptitiously out the door and then whispered: "Wehicles is for white people."

I laughed. All the drivers were white. During the morning shuttles, the radio was a flashpoint for tension. Black people wanted Soul on one end of the FM dial, while the white people liked Rock down the other end. I tuned to Soul going downtown, and then Rock after the van had emptied. I hushed the occasional impertinent request for Rock on the downtown leg with a soft, "Oh, I want to hear this one," regardless of what was playing, and then conveniently forgot the request soon after. Sometimes I patiently dialed in a baseball game on the AM band. Baseball was like a balm for the tension caused by the radio.

"That's true," I said. "Why are all the drivers white?"

"Brothers don't need a license," Keith said. He cut his eyes toward the hallway outside the office and kept his voice low.

I nodded as if this made sense. But I couldn't imagine anyone not having a driver's license, much less an entire race without a license. Aaron explained that public transportation in New York City was so good, you didn't need a license unless you lived in a suburb. The few white people at Rockford other than me were from Staten Island, The Rockaways, or Throggs Neck. Mostly the white people were older, had lost their jobs, lost their health insurance, and then succumbed to some sort of addiction, typically crack. Rockford was the end of the line—free drug treatment.

*   *   *

Summertime—hotter. I got an official letter from the New York City Office of Child Support. I had a hearing in a few weeks.

Showing up on the appointed day, I found the courthouse crowded and loud. Mothers held crying infants to their breasts. Tile floors, crowded wooden benches, impossibly high ceilings, and dusty light fixtures. I met a thin lawyer with a soulful expression and an armful of manila file folders. He asked my name, and then shuffled through his paperwork.

"Welfare?" He studied my file.

I nodded. As we waited outside the courtroom, the heavy wooden doors suddenly burst open. A young man exploded into the lobby, swearing loudly, his face red, wet, and swollen.

"Bitch, fucking bitch!" he screamed. "Goddamn fucking bitch!" A large vein throbbed on the young man's forehead, and his eyes bulged from his face. Were he not in such obvious distress, it would have been comic.

He continued to curse loudly even as a small man in a suit helped him toward the courtroom exit. The man in the suit spoke slowly and evenly, trying his best to defuse the situation. A number of uniformed men looked sternly in the young man's direction. The small man in the suit waved the police off and herded his man out of the court.

"We're up," my lawyer said.

As I entered the courtroom, I saw the judge sitting theatrically high on the other side of the room. She was visibly upset—her brows knitted together, and speaking sharply and with much irritation to the clerks in the room—but she still showed much better composure than her last case. One of the clerks read my name. Turning her attention to my case, the judge scowled at the paperwork before her for a long time. My lawyer hesitantly spoke into the microphone on our side of the room, "He's below the line, Your Honor."

"I can read," she sniped. She asked me to explain myself and I did the best I could. She grunted and set the monthly support to a nominal cost.

Although the amount was low, I reflected uncomfortably that I couldn't pay it. And the thought of it accruing, perhaps accumulating penalties, as I languished in treatment stepped up my discomfort. I whispered as much to my lawyer. He looked surprised. But before he could say anything, the judge asked if I had something to add. I edged up to the microphone to tell her my concern.

Out of the side of his mouth, my lawyer whispered, "*Shut up.*" I could hear the urgency in his voice.

The judge stared down at me over her glasses. My lawyer kept his eyes straight ahead.

"No ma'am," I said.

She rapped her gavel and put the matter to rest. Outside the courtroom, I asked my lawyer again how I was going to pay for the child support. He laughed at me with what seemed like genuine amusement. "You'll think of something," he said.

* * *

During the humid summer that followed, I liked to hang out with Aaron, especially on weekends. Each week at Rockford, there was a Sunday celebration: families brought home-cooked meals, girlfriends appeared in tight jeans and teased hair, and sons mended family ties.

Aaron and I never participated.

He had a girlfriend in Manhattan, but she was ignoring him while he was in treatment. I occasionally wrote my mother carefully composed letters that never asked for anything, or even posed any questions she might feel compelled to answer. I didn't want to pressure her. In prior treatment experiences, I had pushed for the organized reconciliation, the weekend visits. I couldn't imagine going through all that again.

As the summer wore on, counselors began to disappear, with little explanation for their absence. Juan was gone. Rick was gone. A few others were gone. Aaron pointed out that they had actually relapsed and then had to be let go. When I suggested they might have gotten better jobs, Aaron laughed. He was shrewd.

"They're junkies," he said. "You can tell they're in trouble, if their caseload suddenly gets cut." This appeared to be true.

Miguel, who had pale yellow where the whites of his eyes should have been, had his caseload cut to a third of what it once had been. A few days later, he took his remaining charges into the courtyard, and then nodded off in his folding chair during group. One-by-one his clients stood, folded their chairs and then wandered off, until only Miguel was left in the courtyard, his chin upon his chest. News of the counselors' relapses terrified me. It was exactly the kind of thing I could see myself doing.

One Sunday evening in the cafeteria, Aaron mentioned his girlfriend had been to visit him. "Here?" I asked, surprised. I was eagerly forking my way through a pile of rice and beans. Last I had heard about Aaron's girlfriend, she had folded up his diploma from NYU and sent it to him in a No. 10 envelope. I asked him about the creased diploma.

"Bitch," he said, grinning. "But it looks like we're back together."

"Back together?" I asked.

I laid my fork down.

"I'm going to split after dinner," he said. I nodded, my disappointment quickly consuming me. I toyed with my fork. Aaron kept eating. Trying to rally, I encouraged him to stay, to finish his treatment, to address his addiction.

He lowered his fork and grinned at me. "Here?" he laughed. He gave me his new address and phone number, and then he was gone.

* * *

Trains shrieked through Grand Concourse station at 149th Street. Mike and a few others stood in a small group on the platform, waiting for the train. We were on our way to sign up for a job training program in the South Bronx.

I leaned against one of the platform stanchions, lost in thought. As summer came to a close, we had to get jobs, find apartments, and make concrete plans to move out of the facility. This was my chief dilemma.

I was determined to move back to Pennsylvania, even though the mere thought of doing so gave me a knot in my stomach. I wanted to go home. To get out of New York City. But to make that kind of transition, I'd need support. I'd need somewhere to live while I looked for a job. And I'd need food and shelter as I saved up for an apartment. And that's not even considering the intangibles of recovery, like depression, coping with the lack of companionship, and the requirement for constant encouragement that only the truly needy can hope to understand. Most guys would turn to their family for this kind of support. Only problem was, I'd burned those bridges, rebuilt them, then burned them all down again. More than once. My family would be crazy to take a big risk with me. I snorted bitterly at my own intractable predicament. Like Dorothy in *The Wizard of Oz*, I just wanted to go home. But more and more, home was looking like a mirage, an unreachable dream.

"Timmy," Mike shouted. He was right in my face, but I hadn't noticed until he raised his voice. "What's wrong with you?"

"S'up?" I asked.

"You can't stand on the platform like that," Mike said.

"Like what," I asked, confused. I looked down at myself: zipper up, sneakers tied. I seemed okay.

"All lost," Mike said. The others circled around me, nodding their heads. "Someone see you standing like that," Mike said. "You going to get robbed. Or punched."

I laughed. "I got stuff on my mind, man."

"Look, you always got to be scanning, scanning." Mike looked to the left, then to the right. Taking his time, he folded his arms across his chest. "You got to be on guard." He looked completely at ease, the lord of all he surveyed. "You try," he said.

"What are we looking for," I asked.

Everyone chuckled. Mike shook his head in mock disgust. "You looking for trouble, girls, anything." Mike laughed.

I looked to the left, then to the right. I felt awkward, uncomfortable.

"Good, good. That's it," Mike said. "Now check the package."

"The package?" I asked.

More chuckling.

"The package," Mike said. He took a step back and scanned the platform to his left. As he turned his head to the right, he reached down and briefly touched his groin. "Check the package."

I laughed. I had seen others do that gesture a thousand times but had never done it myself. "Why you doing that?" I asked.

"Why?" Mike rolled his eyes. "You got to make sure the package intact," Mike said. "Everything solid."

Trying to duplicate the gesture, I made everyone groan with disappointment. "No, no, no," Mike said. "You adjusting yourself. If you need an adjustment, go to the bathroom."

I laughed, embarrassed.

"Just a quick check," Mike said. He narrowed his eyes and touched his groin. I laughed at how easily he slipped in and out of his hard veneer.

Mike insisted I try a dozen more times. Everyone critiqued my stance, offered suggestions, and little signature moves of their own. I started getting into it. We were all getting into it, styling on the platform: sniffing, looking hard, and touching our groins. When the crowded train pulled up, we filed into the car in a good mood, dispersing to the few vacant spots.

The train doors slid closed and the car pulled out of the station. As the movement of the train jostled my body, I gripped the handrail tighter. Soon my mind wandered back to how I could get myself back to Pennsylvania. Back *home*.

Looking across the car, I found Mike staring at me. When our eyes met, he soundlessly mouthed the word, "*Package*."

* * *

"If you go back to Pennsylvania," Carter was saying, "you won't have any support." A murmur of assent rose up from our little group; a small ring gathered in the empty cafeteria. Tonight was my night.

I nodded.

"You won't be able to attend outpatient aftercare at Rockford."

I inhaled deeply.

"You won't have your peer group to rely upon."

Sweat beading on his forehead, Carter leaned forward in his chair. As he spoke, he used his fingers to tick off all the reasons he felt my return to Pennsylvania was a bad idea. He was on his thumb.

We had been in group for an hour, most of the time focused on me. I knew the trick to getting through a group like this was to look each man in the eye. Listen. Never cross your arms or legs. Appear open, attentive, receptive.

As Carter leaned back in his seat and wiped his forehead with his sleeve, I nodded my head. He appeared to be finished. Clearing my throat, I briefly summarized what Carter, and then each man before him, had said over the past hour. I spoke clearly. Looked each man in the eye. I acknowledged particularly perceptive points. When I was finished, I paused.

Leaning forward, I addressed the entire group.

"Never-" I said, pausing, looking around the room, "the-less."

There was silence for a beat. As the group put together what I had just said, groans rose up from our little ring of chairs.

"I am not staying in New York City after treatment," I continued. "That would be foolish."

Mild cursing started. Someone said, "Fuck him. Send his hillbilly ass back to Pennsylvania." I felt amused, but I did not grin, for I did not want to risk being misunderstood on this matter.

Terrance Tyson sighed. I thought he was going to curse me out, or rally one last argument to change my mind, but instead he chuckled. "You one stubborn motherfucker," he said. Somehow he made it sound endearing.

I shrugged.

Looking at his watch, Terrance closed the group.

* * *

At the front of the classroom, Mr. Parker looked uncomfortable in his collar and tie. He wore his hair in a short, irregular afro, speckled with grey. He stammered when he spoke.

Mike sat to my left, his long legs folded under the desk. Mr. Parker had wobbly hands, which he tried to hide by stuffing them in his pants pockets. New to teaching, he admitted being unfamiliar with the course he was presenting.

Pointing to a small pile of lumber in the corner of the room, Mr. Parker asked us to build the framework for a wall with a window and then excused himself. We pushed all the chairs and desks to the walls.

Pablo had a quick smile and curly dark hair. He wasn't a client at Rockford, but had signed up for this Bronx County training program. Pablo and Mike were natural leaders, taking charge of our little group as everyone started sorting the wood in the lumber pile. The studs were already cut, so assembling the wall was more puzzle then building project. The ring of our hammers broke the early morning quiet.

When Mr. Parker came back into the room, we were raising the wall. He leaned over my shoulder to get a look at what we were doing, and I could smell the pungent odor of whiskey.

"Jesus," I said, waving my hand in front of my face.

Mr. Parker grinned and moved to the center of our group. He extolled our building prowess. Mike and Pablo stood by the little pile of lumber. Everyone stopped building and looked at the unfinished wall we had just raised. Mr. Parker continued to praise our work. Mike offered Mr. Parker a piece of gum and suggested it was time for morning break. Mr. Parker agreed.

Pablo and I followed Mike to a playground across the street from the school. As we entered the yard, Mike wheeled around and said: "We have to help Mr. Parker."

"He's an alcoholic," I groaned. "A loser."

"What the fuck are you?" Mike's tone was sharp.

I rolled my eyes.

The only alcoholic I had ever known had been Maryanne's father, who had died a nasty death from his own out-of-control drinking. I had never been much of a drinker myself and had a hard time seeing my own limitations reflected in the cravings of an alcoholic.

After morning break, we finished building the framework for the wall and then attached sheets of drywall. Mr. Parker said he didn't know how to do the drywall seams, but I told Mike I knew how to tape. I spread the joint compound over the seams, laid down the tape, and then wiped it clean. Everyone cheered.

When we broke for lunch, Mike poked his head into the administrator's office. I went to the swing to eat, and Pablo sat on the merry-go-round. Mike came over in high spirits. He said he had put in a good word for Mr. Parker with the program administrators. Adjusting his utility belt and hammer, he said he felt like a superhero.

Mike said all his friends in Brooklyn called him Black. "But in the Bronx," he said, "I'm Blackman." Pablo laughed and said he was Blackman's trusty sidekick, Puerto Rican Bird.

I chuckled. Mike looked at me expectantly, but I couldn't come up with my own nickname. It wouldn't be right.

"You be Rem Ram," Mike said.

"Rem Ram?" I asked.

"You're an artist," Mike said. "Look what you did with that tape."

"You mean like Rembrandt?" I asked.

"You can go old school, if you want. . ." Mike chuckled.

I was a sucker for a nickname and it felt good to get one from Mike. He might have been five years younger than me, but Mike felt like an older brother. Once, a few months earlier, when we were riding the Lexington Avenue line back to Rockford, Mike had asked me to follow him between the cars. I did, and we stood on the short lip outside the cabin as the train raced north, me looking expectantly at Mike and him motioning for me to be patient. I perched next to him on the precarious ledge of the rocketing car, looking down at the tracks speeding past in a blur beneath my feet, letting the damp tunnel air rush over my face, feeling the car pitch to-and-fro, and listening to the clickety-clack of the tracks. The car thundered from the tunnel and we were suddenly bathed in warm sunshine and fresh air. Mike grinned at me and craned to put his whole head into the sunshine beaming down between the cars. A few minutes later, he pointed to the left, and we saw the sudden emerald green of Yankee Stadium's outfield, glimmering like some hidden verdant treasure as we rushed to the Mount Eden Avenue station.

Mike showed me things in a way I wasn't used to seeing.

I really liked Mike.

When we got back to class, Mike learned that Mr. Parker had been reprimanded over lunch for using the wrong type of drywall for our class project. We had used the green drywall, but we were supposed to have used the white. Mike grew sullen.

During afternoon break, we hung out in the stairwell together, smoking cigarettes. "Once again," I said, "a good man may lose his job over color."

Mike looked sternly at me. "Don't even joke like that," he said. "You have no idea. That's not funny."

Mike went on about Mr. Parker, but I didn't catch much of what he said. I felt ashamed. Mike had never scolded me for saying stupid things before. I wanted to say something to make up for it, but I had no idea what to say. My mouth started moving and, like an idiot, I found myself repeating the exact same thing I had just said, the thing Mike had warned me not to say again.

"Once again," I said, "a good man may lose his job because of color."

"I just told you about that," Mike said. "The *fuck* . . ." Shaking his head, he exhaled noisily. He narrowed his eyes and scowled at me.

The atmosphere in the stairwell grew tense.

Looking down at my shoes, I thought he might hit me. I half-hoped he would. I didn't deserve a friend like Mike.

Finally, Mike stood up and shook his head. "Shit," he sighed. "You're deep."

Mike went back to the classroom. I followed. Mr. Parker droned on for the rest of the afternoon and I found it hard to pay attention. Instead of learning how to build walls, I should have been learning how to build friendships. I felt useless. When I walked to the train after class, I hung back from Mike and Pablo.

After half a block, Mike looked over his shoulder and spied me lagging. "Rem Ram," he said. "Get your ass up here."

* * *

October brought an Indian summer. To celebrate, Rockford organized an impromptu cookout. I watched as Terrance and the others prepared the grill, a 55-gallon drum cut in half longways. Examining the grill, I pricked my index finger on its ragged edge.

Terrance looked at the wound, which was already starting to swell, then sent me to the ER. "That grill been around since World War II," he said. "You better get yourself checked."

Sitting in the crowded lobby at Bronx Lebanon Hospital, I watched my injured hand develop a dark red welt above one of the veins in my wrist. After an hour, I was still waiting and the welt had moved up my arm, past the elbow, along the same vein. I pointed this out to the hospital staff and heard my name called a few minutes later. Moments after that, I was led to a bed.

A small, disheveled, Asian doctor and a heavyset nurse in white approached me as I sat on the bed. The little man silently poked my finger with an instrument and looked at my arm. Rattling off something to the nurse in a language I couldn't follow, he put his back to me, took my hand under his arm, and adjusted his footing.

The nurse said, "He say this going to hurt."

At the word "hurt," I grew alarmed and tried to extricate my hand. The doctor looked over his shoulder and spoke again to the nurse, casting a glance at me. I narrowed my eyes, but left my hand under his arm.

"He say this the only way," the nurse said.

I looked at her in disbelief.

"Don't worry," she said. "We give you something for pain."

When she said "something for pain," my ears perked up. I knew then I'd let the doctor work on me, but I didn't want to appear too eager, so I asked a few more questions, to make it look as if I were considering all the options.

The nurse said that I had a staph infection and would likely need to remain in the hospital for a few days. I considered asking for more details about the *something for pain*, but the doctor was waiting, instrument in hand.

I nodded to the little doctor. "G' head," I said.

He broke open the wound and cleaned it out.

Within an hour I had been admitted to a room. To my great disappointment, however, the promised pain medication was two tablets of acetaminophen with codeine in a little paper cup.

I scowled at the nurse, and she said we could try something stronger if there was still more pain. I sighed and took the medicine.

I was in the room alone. You had to pay a fee to get TV and I had no money. My hand throbbed but I could feel the drugs faintly at the back of my head. When the nurse came in to ask how I was doing, I waved her off. I just wanted to enjoy the codeine tickling the back of my head.

I was allowed another dose of pain medication every four hours. I kept on top of the staff and didn't tolerate lateness. If I wanted to smoke a cigarette, I had to go down the hall. I put off the walk as long as I could so as not to disturb my high.

On the morning of the second day, I thought again about how I might get back to Pennsylvania. In all the excitement, I realized I hadn't given Pennsylvania any thought for two entire days. Remembering the familiar problem, I felt as if I were greeting an old friend. The small amount of codeine had emboldened me, and I realized with startling clarity this one simple fact: It was ridiculous for me to consider returning to Pennsylvania after treatment for all the reasons my counselors and peers had been listing over the last few months.

My best chance at recovery would be to stay in New York City and continue doing what I was already doing. I would have to get a job and find a place to live. As soon as I thought about living in New York, I felt an immense sense of relief. When I felt the relief, I knew I was on the right track. Something clicked. For the rest of the morning, I turned it around and around in my mind. I felt a little humiliation for having been so stubborn the last six months. And I was not looking forward to recanting in group. But I was also unmistakably excited. I could do it; I could actually live in New York City. Instead of the nagging fear, I realized I had an opportunity here to do something I might otherwise never have been able to accomplish. I would have the support of the entire facility as I looked for work and an apartment. For the first time in months, I felt genuinely hopeful.

At one point, the on-duty nurse came into my room. "Your hand feeling better, I see," she said. Her tone seemed authoritative. We were hours from my next dose of pain medication.

"Why you say that?" I asked.

She nodded toward my hand.

I hadn't realized it, but I had both my hands tucked behind my head. Pulling my bandaged hand out, I looked at it with such surprise the nurse started to chuckle. I reluctantly admitted the throbbing had indeed gone away.

A day later, I was back at Rockford.

In a counseling session soon after, Ramon chided me about getting a three-day vacation. I told him about the codeine and asked if I would have to do anything—say, extend my time in treatment—for having taken it.

"How do you feel?" he asked.

"Fine," I said. I held up my hand and worked my injured finger.

"No," he laughed. "I mean, do you feel obsessed to use more drugs?"

"No," I said. "Not at all." I hadn't even considered it.

He told me not to worry. The codeine had been for a legitimate medical purpose. He reminded me to declare it if I got selected for a random urine analysis.

"Shit," he chuckled. "Three days off *and codeine*? Pfffffft. Somebody give me a knife," he mugged. "I'm going to cut my hand right now."

I felt too embarrassed to tell Ramon about the awareness I'd had about me living in New York. However, I savored the irony of a recovering heroin addict needing a tiny bit of opiate to get on the right track. I had been trying to solve the riddle of how to get back to Pennsylvania for so long, it felt good to let it all go. I knew that staying in New York City was my best good hope.

I had found my way home. And home wasn't in Pennsylvania.

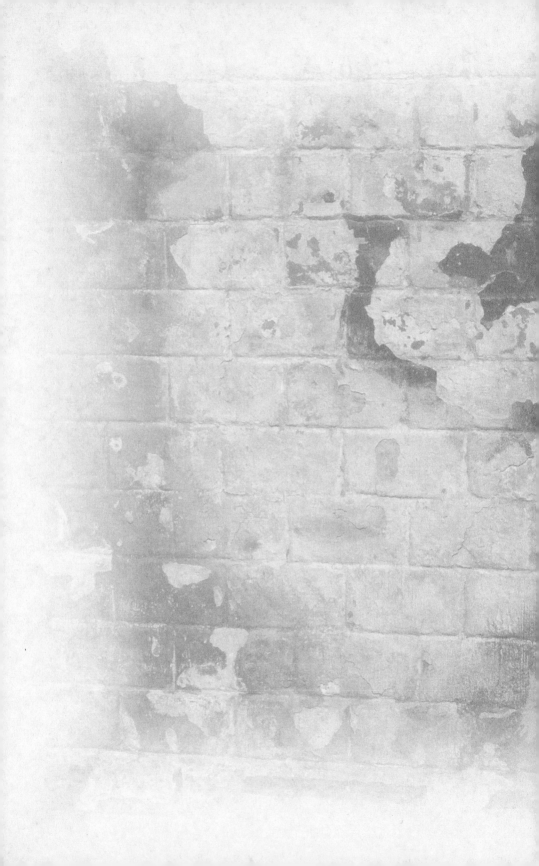

CHAPTER 3

FAITH

Entering Rockford's lobby, I heard shouts and laughter from the main hall.

I had spent the afternoon looking for work in Manhattan, enjoying the brisk fall weather and the heady experience of being out of the facility unescorted for the first time in almost a year. To hear shouting and laughter from the main hall was unusual. Turning the corner, I found James, swearing and chuckling with Rockford's second-in-command, the wheelchair-bound Franklin.

Rumor held that Franklin had been paralyzed in a shootout when he was still using drugs. Both Franklin and James were former addicts who had come through treatment at Rockford, taken jobs as counselors, and then risen to positions of authority. The only people with more clout seemed to be the board members, the old men and women with white hair in meticulously pressed suits and dresses, who occasionally came to press events or graduation functions.

"Driver, driver," Franklin barked from his chair. Turning to James, he said, "Time to take my black ass home."

As he waited for the driver and escort to emerge from the Vehicles Office, Franklin continued a too-loud conversation with James. I could tell they had both been drinking. In other facilities, even moderate drinking would have been considered a relapse. Here it was just another privilege to earn, much like looking for work or moving out of the facility.

I still felt certain my best hope was to remain in New York City, but my reservations about Rockford only seemed to grow stronger with time.

*   *   *

Manhattan, nighttime. Late October.

I was returning to the facility from an evening job interview at Grand Central. The position was for maintaining indoor plants in Manhattan atriums during the middle of the night. Graveyard shift.

I decided to hit a recovery meeting before returning to Rockford. To save a subway token, I strode almost forty blocks uptown to a church on the Upper East Side that hosted round-the-clock meetings for alcoholics. I knew heroin addicts who had stopped using heroin by going to meetings for alcoholics, but I wasn't certain about my own chances of finding recovery this way. If nothing else, I took comfort in the fact that I was implicitly offering a big "fuck you" to James and Franklin by attending a meeting for alcoholics. Racing down the concrete stairs, I stepped into the basement just as the meeting began. There were less than a dozen people, but this seemed crowded for a weekday at 10:00 p.m.

Over time, certain institutions can begin to lose their character and look depressingly similar—think jail cells, the offices of social workers, or cheap hotel rooms. This room had metal folding chairs and walls filled with signs of positive aphorism ("Keep Coming Back" and "One Day at a Time"). The leader introduced a humorless speaker, who looked about twenty years older than me and immediately began an earnest discussion of God. What he said sounded familiar in the same way the room looked familiar— characterless, uniform, and grim.

One Old Testament definition of faith is *being sure of what we hope for and certain of what we do not see*. I had close to a year of abstinence but very little confidence in my own abilities, or really even the ability of any recovery program or drug treatment facility to help me to continue to remain abstinent. One thing that I did have absolute confidence in was something that I couldn't see—namely my addiction to heroin, my seemingly limitless capacity to turn my life upside down, which I had proven to myself time and time again.

Looking around the room, I spied a face I knew all too well: Chopper Cassidy, who had died of a drug overdose in Steelton ten years ago. While he was alive, I'd only known him in the way that troublemakers know one another in a small town. Once, he had sold me four phony Quaaludes, at four dollars apiece. Outweighing me as he did by twenty-five pounds, there was little I could do but (literally) eat the loss.

In death, however, we had become much closer.

He sat in one of the steel folding chairs, grinning and listening to the speaker talk about God. Wearing Chuck Taylor All-Stars and a threadbare denim jacket, Chopper Cassidy looked more or less the same as he did ten years ago. Each time he showed up, I compared the ways in which we were different. I'd now passed him in age. I'd put on enough weight of my own that his great bulk seemed less threatening. I could even remember a time when all of us wore Chuck Taylors. Sometimes the most painful realizations in life are the most obvious. The worst part about the occasional appearance from Chopper Cassidy was that I understood I wasn't all that different from him.

Not really. Not in any meaningful way.

Chopper Cassidy sat next to a young woman who listened attentively to the speaker. Leaning his great bulk over her, he glimpsed down her shirt.

She looked right through him.

I turned my gaze to the wall. I tried to listen to the speaker, but his voice faded to a dull monotone. Unable to stop myself, I stole another glimpse over my shoulder.

Fishing a pickle from a businessman's deli sandwich, Chopper Cassidy sniffed it, then flung it across the room. The businessman took a bite of his sandwich and set it on his lap to clap for the speaker.

Soon everyone began clapping. The speaker had finished.

I turned in my seat and began to clap, too. I sat up straighter and kept my eyes facing toward the front of the room.

There was one important difference between Chopper Cassidy and me.

I wasn't dead.

Yet.

When the leader of the meeting asked if anyone needed a sponsor, I raised my hand. After the meeting, the leader gave me the phone number of a man named Roger, who had specifically asked to help someone new.

I put Roger's phone number in my pocket.

When I looked for Chopper Cassidy again, he was gone. I helped put the folding chairs away and then hurried through the cold night air to the train station and Rockford.

*   *   *

Getting a job was easier than I'd expected.

The day after Chopper Cassidy appeared at the meeting, a girl from the plant maintenance company with which I had interviewed the previous night called and offered me a position on the atrium crew. And just like that, I was working.

Each night I traveled from Rockford to various locations in Manhattan, to work on a three-man crew.

My boss possessed a Ph.D. in Agriculture, and drove the company truck in from New Jersey every night. He smoked a pipe and had long wavy hair that he furtively admired in any reflective surface. His intellectual curiosity seemed limitless, but he indulged himself too much to be of much help to the crew. He would do things like stretch out on the floor nearby a planter box, watching for hours to learn how a community of aphids organized themselves to solve certain logistical issues. We all knew about his degree because he told us. He constantly found ways to remind us about his degree. He once bragged, "My goal is to get you to a point where you can think exactly like me."

The crew lieutenant was Jamir, who lived somewhere in Manhattan and spoke with a thick Indian accent. Five years older than me, with a stout belly, Jamir smoked thin brown cigarettes and knew a lot about tropical plants.

We bonded over our dislike for the Ph.D.

In Pennsylvania, I had worked for several nurseries where we dug holes with backhoes and used our muddy boots to tamp roots. Here the work was much different, the plants exotic and delicate. I dusted, trimmed, and watered. Late at night, my footsteps echoed eerily in the soaring atrium spaces.

From a payphone in Trump Tower, I called my brand-new recovery sponsor, whom I had not even met yet. Roger was pleasant, but those first few phone calls were uncomfortable. He was, after all, an alcoholic. He gave me all of his contact numbers: a work number, a number to a mobile phone the size and weight of a paving brick, even multiple weekend numbers in Vermont. Drug dealers didn't have so many phone numbers. Roger said to call whenever I wanted, but if it was after 10:00 p.m., the call had to be urgent. I always tried to call at the start of my shift. He suggested I try attending ninety meetings in ninety days—the old "90-in-90." I told him I would.

Every night the Ph.D. told me what to do. I would get started, but then I always ran the Ph.D.'s instructions past Jamir for review. The Ph.D. was smart, but Jamir kept the work running smoothly. After work, I went to an early morning recovery meeting and then back to Rockford. Eventually I told Jamir I was in rehab, but never would I entrust this information to the Ph.D.

Soon there was a company-wide effort to recruit extra hands to set up Christmas decorations. For the promise of time-and-a-half, I eagerly signed up. Every account needed some combination of red and white poinsettias, acres and acres of tiny white lights, and bough upon bough of holly.

During the first day of overtime, I met Rachel, a girl from the front office who had a soft chin and delicate overbite. You could tell she didn't think much of her looks, but this shyness just made her that much more appealing. I felt confident around her. She had moved east from Arizona with a degree in agriculture and was on her own for the holidays.

I was circumspect about my personal information. "I live up in the Bronx," I said, trying to affect a street wisdom I hadn't really earned. "Been here almost a year."

By the end of the holiday weekend, I mustered the courage to ask her out.

"Would you like to go out with me? Would that make you happy?" In treatment we'd been drilled on communicating clearly with others, and I wondered if I'd come on too strong.

But Rachel just seemed pleasantly surprised by my straightforwardness. "I would like that," she said. "Yes."

* * *

With the new job came new privileges. I moved into a special wing at Rockford with others who had jobs. We got weekend passes and more freedom to come and go.

One evening, I was waiting my turn to use the pay phone in the hall to call Roger.

"Timmy," Mickey said. "Check this out, dude."

Mickey was twenty years older than me. He wore thick glasses and kept his wavy gray hair meticulously oiled and combed. A career criminal, he had spent most of his life in prison. His age gave him a certain gravitas the other clients lacked. He struck me as being wise. Once I overheard him tell a story about how he realized he had to change his life's trajectory. During his final incarceration, a young inmate had brushed past him and without any malice said, 'Excuse me, Pop.' As Mickey recounted this story, he shook his fist and repeated, "Pop," with a rueful chuckle. He felt insulted. But then he realized the inmate hadn't intended to offend him. His youth really had slipped away.

Standing next to me, he gestured with his hands as he spoke. "We split the cost of an apartment," he said, "we can get the hell outta here."

As soon as he said it, I realized it made sense.

I told Mickey to let me think about it, but I was mostly decided.

I got on the phone to Roger. I had been unable to attend meetings each day during the holiday overtime and now I felt terrible. I had ruined my 90-in-90. I wanted everything to go perfectly, but here I was not even out of treatment, and already I was making compromises.

"Well, I messed up," I said into the phone.

"You drank?" Roger asked. "I don't understand."

"No, no, no." I said, "Not that bad. I just missed a few meetings."

I was sure Roger was going to tell me to start over from the beginning, like one of those computer games where you had to do everything perfectly to advance to the next level. That's what most sponsors I'd had in the past would've said. I felt a little depressed, mildly defeated. But I also felt determined to make a good effort at recovery.

"I still don't understand," Roger said. "Can you just go to another one? See if you can squeeze in two on a single day."

"Can I do that?" I asked.

"Hell, yeah!" Roger laughed. "You know what happens when you finally go to ninety meetings in ninety days?" Not waiting for me to answer, he said, "You go to ninety-one."

I laughed. I could see I was going to like this guy.

* * *

Rachel and I started dating.

One weekend we went to a movie and then stomped around Manhattan, enjoying the holiday decorations. We ended up in New Jersey at her apartment, which she shared with a cat that sent me into fits of uncontrolled sneezing. I felt anxious that first night. I could tell Rachel was a nice girl, from a good family. I hadn't gone out with a nice girl since my wife had left me. For the last few years, intimacy mostly meant renting a stack of porn tapes and a weekend of casual sex. I had never even had sex without being a little stoned or drunk. Fortunately, my frenzied sneezing helped take my mind off my fears. When it finally happened, having sex with a clear head was better than I could have imagined.

After that first night at Rachel's apartment, we dispensed with the pretense of dates in Manhattan, and I came directly to her apartment on the following weekends. I agonized over how much to tell her about my situation, finally deciding to reveal everything. She didn't seem to mind. We spent our days in a tangle of sheets on her fold-out couch.

Rachel was popular in the company, and soon I noticed my stock rising, too. We attended a holiday party together and sat at a table with the owner and his wife. I liked the attention, but it also made me a little uncomfortable.

One night I had Rachel take me to her neighborhood video store.

"Got any porn?" I asked the middle-aged clerk. From the corner of my eye, I saw Rachel cringe. Wordlessly the clerk indicated a small room behind a pair of swinging saloon-type doors. Rachel said she had never even noticed this part of the store before.

I told her I believed her.

*　*　*

After Christmas, Jamir took over the night crew. The Ph.D. had somehow got himself transferred back to dayshift in New Jersey.

This should have been great, but it went downhill fast. We had never really counted on the Ph.D. to do much work, but now Jamir and I were completing our normal tasks, as well as tasks that had long been on the backlog for want of additional manpower. Jamir grew demanding. Worse, all the shortcuts that he had taught me were now suddenly forbidden. Without the Ph.D. to rail on, it turned out we didn't have much in common.

Our friendship began to fade.

During my evening phone calls with Roger, I complained bitterly about Jamir night after night. One evening, I had myself going pretty good describing the latest changes that Jamir had forced upon me. Roger interrupted.

"Maybe you should pray for him," Roger said. "You ever think of that?"

"Pray for Jamir?" I said. "*Jamir?*"

Twisting my face, I held the phone about a foot from my ear and stared at the receiver in my hand. I barked, "Are you even listening?"

I was so distraught, I had to remind myself to put the phone back to my ear so the conversation could continue. Roger was chuckling. He assured me he was listening. He said getting too angry posed a risk to people in recovery. Roger had a smooth, silky voice, like a pool of maple syrup filling a breakfast plate. More than anything else, the sound of his voice, the warm cadence of it, softened my feelings.

At meetings, I had heard the business about praying for the people who pissed you off. To me, it sounded corny, and I told Roger as much.

"You don't have to do it," he said. "Just be careful about getting too angry."

"That sounds ominous," I said.

Roger laughed. He assured me he didn't mean it as a threat. "Pay attention to your feelings," he said. "And don't drink."

*   *   *

I came home from work one morning, and Mickey asked if I wanted to go check out an apartment on the other side of the Bronx.

"Dude," Mickey said. "This is it."

We rode downtown to the Grand Concourse, and then switched to an uptown train. When we came down from the elevated station at Pelham Parkway, I thought we were in another city. There were wide, inviting streets without any trash. Tall oaks and thick maples dotted the sidewalks in every direction, their naked branches soaring in a cloudless sky. The median between the parkway's eastbound and westbound lanes held a swath of grass so wide it looked like rolling pasture.

Mickey led the way to a two-story duplex not far from the train.

The landlord was a sturdy old man with a shock of white hair and a craggy face. He led us upstairs and waited patiently as we poked around. Four rooms with gleaming hardwood floors and thick, ornate moldings on doors and ceilings. A small kitchen and a big bathroom.

Mickey looked disappointed.

He opened the oven and refrigerator. Flushed the toilet and then let the spigots run hot. He paced the hall and inspected all the closets. Mickey spoke softly with the landlord for a few minutes and then asked if I were ready to go.

I assumed Mickey didn't like the place and that was fine with me. Given a little more time, I was sure we'd find something even better. Mickey told the landlord he would call, and we headed back toward the train.

As we turned the corner, Mickey came alive. His face sparkled.

"Dude," Mickey said, "that place is a beauty."

"You liked it?" I asked.

"You didn't," Mickey said.

I shrugged. "It's fine," I said. "I just thought we might look a little longer, see if something better turned up."

Mickey assured me we would find nothing better. He seemed irritated. He had a job in the mail room at Jacobi Hospital and pointed out that this apartment was within easy walking distance. We worked out the financials and discovered we could do it, but only if we pooled our money. As we boarded our train, I agreed to move forward.

Mickey grew ecstatic. His face lit up.

"Dude," he laughed. Clapping me on the back, he said, "You're going to have a New York City address."

"It's not funny," I snapped, the anger in my voice surprising both him and me.

"You think this is all a big joke, but it's not." I gripped the handrail of the train as it rocked along.

"Anything could happen," I said. "You can never really know how things will turn out. Things might be fine one minute, but then the next, you find yourself in the gutter."

Mickey kept his seat but looked at me curiously.

I went on like this, ranting, finger-wagging. I have no idea what else I said, but when I finished, I slumped down into the seat, exhausted by the outpouring of emotion. My head felt light, and a clammy feeling grew under my arms.

We rode silently the rest of the way, the train swaying our bodies.

Eventually we pulled into a station, and I had to hold myself to keep from sliding into Mickey. I felt too embarrassed to look at him. When we pulled out of the station, I felt his hand lightly on my shoulder.

"Dude," Mickey said softly. "You okay?"

* * *

I broke it off with Rachel.

I didn't want to, but I didn't see any other choice. Things were changing between us, it seemed, and I couldn't be sure how it would all pan out. When I slept over her house—after we had our coffee in the morning—she would rouse me from the bed and want to fold it back into a couch. Instead of watching porn movies until deep into the afternoon, she wanted to take long drives through the New Jersey hills in the cold sunshine. She was most likely trying to take our relationship to a deeper place, but I was never really sure what she saw in me anyway and reacted with cold fear.

I told myself I needed to prioritize my recovery.

I broke up with her from the payphone in the hall at Rockford. I told Rachel I still liked her, but that I wanted us to be friends.

"Okay," she said, her voice sounding small.

I felt terrible. Rachel sounded glum. Crawling into my cot, I had a restless sleep and then rode the train into Manhattan for work.

* * *

"Sound like an anxiety attack," Terrance said.

We were discussing my outburst on the train with Mickey. "People get 'em all the time," he added. "No big deal."

I had never experienced anything like it before and didn't feel comforted. We were in Terrance's office, signing paperwork so I could move out of the facility.

"You break up with that white girl?" Terrance said. It wasn't really a question. He had his head cocked back and was looking at me like he expected me to lie.

I sighed.

"You asshole," Terrance said. He turned back to his paperwork, shaking his head.

I looked at my feet.

He started to lecture me about self-esteem, but I cut him off. If he knew about Rachel, he must know about the recovery meetings for alcoholics. And if he didn't, I figured I ought to tell him, just to get all the bad news out of the way. I didn't see how anything else I could say would disappoint him any more.

Hearing about my involvement with the alcoholic recovery program, Terrance said, "Well, congratulations. That's the first intelligent thing I've heard you say since you arrived in New York. You're going to need all the support you can get."

I was surprised. I asked him about Franklin, James, and the drinking privileges.

"Those guys are old-school," Terrance said. He leaned back in his chair and took a conversational tone with me, and I felt pleased to be in his confidence. "Back in the day, treatment facilities gave drug addicts drinking privileges if you made it through treatment. But guess what?—"

He sat up his chair and spread his arms wide, palm up.

"Most of the motherfuckers relapsed!"

Terrance settled back in his seat. "Now times have changed. Recovery is hard. Trust me—drinking won't improve your chances."

"I don't drink," he said. He looked me in the eye.

I sat with this revelation for a short time. I felt satisfied that I finally got an honest answer from someone in authority. After a few minutes, I narrowed my eyes. "Why don't Franklin and James try harder to provide a better example?"

Terrance laughed.

He leaned forward across his paper-strewn desk. He was a big man who easily outweighed me by more than thirty pounds. Poking his thick forefinger into my chest, he said: "Keep the focus on yourself."

* * *

I fiddled with a large fig tree in the lobby of Grand Central Station.

I hadn't seen Jamir since coming on my shift, but I knew what we needed to accomplish and kept myself busy.

At Roger's urging, I had given the situation with Jamir some thought. I was pretty sure he had amped the night crew's performance to impress the front office. With the Ph.D. gone, this was Jamir's big chance. What he didn't realize was how hard it was going to be for him to impress those guys in New Jersey. At the holiday party, I had overheard them imitate Jamir's high-pitched, sing-song cadence, even mocking his big belly and tight pants.

Jamir called for me in his familiar cadence. "Tim, Tim!"

I saw him standing in the great doors that open to 42nd Street. He waved me over but kept his position at the door and peered into the street.

Finishing with the tree, I trotted over to Jamir. Today after my shift, I would remove the last of my belongings from Rockford and officially move to the Pelham Parkway apartment. It was a big day.

"Come, come," he said, slipping into the night.

He had a car double-parked in the street with the motor running. He opened the door and motioned for me to get in.

"You bought a car?" I asked.

"Rental," he said. "Come, come."

He drove toward the waterfront in good spirits. I was curious where he had been most of the night, but didn't want to ask and risk wrecking his fine mood. Fiddling with the radio, I looked up to find the glare of oncoming headlights filling the windshield. Horns blared. We were traveling the wrong way up a one way street.

"Jamir!" I said. Pressing my foot into the floorboard, I braced myself for the worst.

"Goddamn," Jamir said. "Goddamn."

He was trying to make a U-turn and muttering to himself. I realized he had been drinking. Amid the shifting, doppler-ized blare of horns all around us, he got the car turned around. We were in an unfamiliar part of Manhattan with big windowless warehouses, the orange glow of high-crime street lights, and long, deep shadows.

"Jamir," I said, fighting for calm. "What are we doing?"

He grinned, a big sloppy smile. "Tonight you finish treatment, yes?" he asked.

I nodded, surprised he had even remembered.

"We celebrate," he said. "Look, look."

In the street ahead, I saw a blur of sequins, a flash of female flesh, short skirts and bikini tops. Prostitutes. Three or four of them had their arms in the air, waving their hands above their heads. I looked at Jamir with confusion and horror. He mistook the look on my face for a question of logistics. "Just climb in the back," he said. "I'll pay."

The light dawned—I'd finished treatment, I was moving into my new apartment and Jamir wanted to get me something, a sort of housewarming gift. I felt alarmed and disgusted, but also a little touched. There was an awful moment where I just didn't know how to respond. Then, from the street, we heard the voices of the women waving their hands.

As one they chanted, "GO HOME! YOU'RE DRUNK! NO SERVICE!"

I laughed, relieved. We'd been flagged.

* * *

My first order of business in the new apartment was to call my mother.

Morning was a good time to be in the apartment; Mickey was at work and I had the place to myself. I sat at the top of the stairwell with the phone in my lap as the sun made big rectangles on the living room floor.

I got my mother on the phone and we made small talk.

For months I had been afraid to think of this exact moment. I would occasionally tantalize myself by imagining this conversation—what I would say, how mom might answer—but then I would quickly stop and try to put it out of my mind; I didn't want to jinx myself. Prior to this, I may have sent her brief notes, but I hadn't called. I didn't want to raise anyone's hopes—least of all my own—until I had a better sense for how things would play out. Dashed hope seemed cruel, something to be avoided at all costs. With the apartment, I felt as if I had something concrete to offer. Hard evidence of success.

Halfway through the conversation, I told her I was sitting in the front hall of my new apartment. I kept my voice casual, not wanting to say anything about feeling hopeless or afraid. I laid it all out for her: the new job, the apartment with Mickey, and the completion of treatment.

"I'm going to live in New York for a while," I said. "See how it goes." The line went silent as my mother considered all this new information.

I rattled on about Joey and my desire to come see him, which so far I had only thought about abstractly. Steelton was a four-hour train ride: I'd need time off, perhaps a long weekend, and a gift, possibly two. I had missed Christmas and his birthday. I avoided saying anything about where I would stay, although I knew this was another thing I had to figure out.

"You can stay here," Mom said. "I have room for you."

"At your house," I said. "I can stay at your house?"

"Sure," Mom said. "I got an open room."

And just like that, I was allowed back in my mother's house again.

* * *

I went to meet Roger for lunch.

I was interested to finally see what he looked like. He worked near Gramercy, on the third floor of a nondescript building. He was twenty years older than me. Tall, with thin hair and a strong jaw, he wore pleated khaki pants and a dark jersey.

He thrust out his hand and smiled.

We walked to a nearby diner in silence. I had spent the night at work and felt sleepy, even a little morose. I slid into the booth and ordered coffee. Roger ordered lunch.

As we started to chat, I wondered aloud how long I would last outside treatment. Roger looked at me quizzically. I said I didn't want to feel this way, but that I was trying to be realistic: I had never been in recovery this long before.

Wiping fried chicken from his fingers and mouth, Roger leaned forward.

"Do you believe that I believe you can recover?" As soon as he said it, he waved his hand in my face and added, "Now listen here! I'm not asking if *you* believe any of this."

He sat back in the booth.

"I'm asking if you believe that *I believe it.*" He jerked his thumb into his chest.

This wasn't a hard question. I knew Roger believed.

"You?" I said. "Sure."

His fist came sailing down and hit the Formica table, jangling all the flatware and water glasses.

"You, my friend," he pointed, "are going to make it!"

He said this with so much gravity and conviction it made me grin.

People at nearby tables raised their heads, but Roger ignored them. He said all you needed was a tiny bit of faith to get by. I leaned back and chuckled.

Roger believed I would make it.

*   *   *

Joey was all grins.

I had just given him a radio-controlled truck with thick knobby tires. It had cost a small fortune, was twice the size of my weekend bag, and meant for a much older child. Every adult who saw this gift and who knew Joey said the exact same thing—he's going to destroy that thing!

The first time I heard this, I took it as criticism, and I felt terrible. I had agonized over selecting the right gift, but was too ashamed to admit I had no idea what sort of gift a four-year-old boy might enjoy. I couldn't imagine coming to see him empty-handed.

Now, sitting in Jack's living room, I watched Joey joyfully tear the truck out of the box, and Maryanne, grinning, predicted it would soon be destroyed.

I shrugged and grinned myself. "Yup," I agreed.

Joey was a little bigger than he had been the last time I had seen him, but he was still just a noodle of a boy, all bony elbows and knees and clipped hair. He liked to play baseball and was turning into quite an athlete, just like my brothers.

He asked me to play catch with him. I didn't see how I could refuse.

We went into the narrow backyard. The late morning air was cold and the sky a dull white. The back of the house was all glass: windows on either side of a storm door, which had two of its own panes of glass. I imagined the look on Jack's face if the ball crashed through any of those windows.

Stationing Joey closest to the house, I tugged on a borrowed glove, and walked toward the alley end of the yard.

"We should switch sides. My Dad says I should always catch on the alley side," Joey said.

I turned to look at the boy and he squinted up at me.

"'Case I miss," he said, nodding toward the glass.

I tried to explain that I had much more confidence in his ability to catch the ball than I did in my own, but he just kept squinting up at me. I pressed on, even tossing him the ball, an easy underhand lob. He caught it effortlessly with a flip of his wrist, but then he looked around uncomfortably.

"We're going to get in trouble," he said. "Big trouble."

I sighed.

We decided our best bet was to go up to the high school field to play. He was a much better catcher than me, and I ran for all the balls I missed. By the time we got back to the house, I felt humiliated, tired, and hungry. Joey didn't seem to notice and he ran into the house ahead of me.

Maryanne offered to make us lunch.

I sat at the table and Joey washed up in the kitchen sink. Looking in the refrigerator, Maryanne told me what she had. I asked for Lebanon bologna, American cheese, lettuce, and yellow mustard.

Joey plopped in the seat next to me and asked for the exact same thing.

As soon as I heard his request, I cut a sideways glance at him. I didn't want to feel anxious, but when I looked down at him and saw his beaming eyes and grinning, happy face, I was terrified.

"You like mustard?" I asked.

It sounded more like an accusation than I had intended, but I couldn't help myself. "And lettuce?" Most people like mayonnaise. Occasionally a guy will put some mustard on a hot dog, but rarely on a sandwich—and never with lettuce.

"Yeah," Joey said. "I like mustard." His voice sounded hesitant, meek. "I like lettuce."

The light in his face dimmed a bit, and I tried my best to backpedal by chuckling, but my mouth was dry and a terrible sound came out.

"You ever have your sandwich like that before?" I asked.

Maryanne turned slowly from the counter with a look of disbelief on her face. "Tim," she said to me. "He wants the same sandwich as you."

I felt embarrassed. "'Course he does," I said. "Of course, of course."

Maryanne looked at me dubiously.

"It's a good sandwich to have," I said to no one in particular.

Joey attacked his lunch. I did the same and Maryanne left us alone. Except for the sound of contented munching, the kitchen grew silent. As Joey ate, I stole looks at his face, trying to imagine what he was seeing when he looked at me.

Later that night, Joey and I went to my mother's house, which was quiet and empty. Joey had come to sleep over. In one of the bedrooms, I made him a nest of blankets on the floor beside the bed where I would sleep.

None of my four brothers or two sisters had come to visit and that was fine with me. They were managing their lives, their families, and their careers. I felt grateful not to have to explain what I had been doing for the past year and a half and even more pleased not to have to lay out any made-up plans for the future. Plus, this way I would get to spend some uninterrupted time with Joey.

Mom invited me to church the next morning. I didn't want to hurt her feelings, but I didn't want to spend four hours at her church service, either. I pointed out that I only had the weekend to see Joey.

To my surprise, Mom agreed my time might be better spent visiting with my boy.

In the past, the deal with my mother had always been that to stay at her house, I had to go to her church. By conceding church, I felt as if she were acknowledging that I was responsible for whatever happened next. This realization was pleasantly satisfying but also made me nervous. I felt as if I had to pull a rabbit from the hat, but I wasn't even sure how the trick worked.

*   *   *

In late spring, I transferred to dayshift.

I had been feeling isolated. Mickey had met a woman his age and spent most of his time with her. When we did see one another, there always seemed to be tension, typically over minor lifestyle issues, such as my disinterest in cleaning or the eagerness with which I devoured his snacks. I offered myself complete absolution for these petty crimes, almost before they even happened, and couldn't understand why I felt so cut off or why there was so much tension. Instead of looking at my part in our disagreements, I blamed working at night and thought the change might do me some good.

But moving to dayshift only added to my stress.

Instead of the big atrium accounts, working dayshift involved visiting smaller offices scattered across Manhattan. A big part of dayshift was to briefly meet with representatives at each account to discuss the health of the plants in their offices. I was terrible at this. I couldn't remember many of the plant names, and I was awful at small talk. I watched helplessly and with increasing desperation as the plants withered into black stalks.

And I refused to order new plants.

I knew the people in the front office gossiped about the different crews' abilities. I felt certain my breakup with Rachel had left me vulnerable to the most vicious of rumors. Soon I began to measure how many paychecks I had left by the condition of the plants in most of my accounts. Surely I would be fired when all that was left of the plants were the rotting hulks of wet root ball.

At one point, Rachel called me. "You can order more plants," she said. "The other techs do it all the time."

I knew she was right, but I also knew I couldn't do the job. Meeting with people. Earnest conversations about plants I couldn't name and for which I had no idea how to care. It all seemed like too much to bear.

In the empty boardrooms of the tall buildings downtown, I tried to ease my anxiety by dialing the 900 number sex lines and talking to anonymous Latino women for hours on end. The beginning of the end came in the heat of August when I started timing my appearance at accounts to coincide with when the representatives would most likely be out or busy. I would race in, rush through the maintenance, and get any receptionist or even janitorial personnel to sign my sheets.

* * *

Moving to dayshift had been a terrible decision. I felt even more isolated than I had on the nightshift.

I called Roger and explained how I was feeling. He asked if I was still going to meetings and if I had made any friends in the program. I was attending meetings but found it difficult to make friends. He offered some suggestions about how to proceed: "Always sit up front," he said. "Say hello to the person on your left and right, and then chat with the speaker after the meeting ends."

I did this for a few weeks and felt incredibly uncomfortable. But learning to socialize seemed like the least I could do to better my situation, so I persevered.

During this time, I would call Roger daily and report in, mostly just to hear his voice. When we ended our calls, he began to say, "I love you," just before we hung up. He would say these words in a very clear manner, making it sound almost formal but never rote or perfunctory. For example, never would he say, "Love ya," or "Lottsa love," or something that might be mistaken for a casual way of ending a conversation. He always said, "I love you," as if he had only recently made up his mind about me and had discovered that it was love. The first time I heard this I was terrified. I held the phone from my ear and looked at the receiver, astonished. What did it mean? I carefully lowered the phone, placing it soundlessly into its cradle, and pretending that I hadn't heard what he had just said.

I didn't tell Mickey or anyone else.

If it were some sort of homosexual come-on, I didn't want to risk the pain and embarrassment of exposure. I had been hustling gay men for sex and money since I was a teen, so I wasn't unfamiliar with homosexuality. But I didn't know what to make of this. It didn't feel sexual. I didn't know how to explain it. Each night at the end of our phone call Roger would say it, sometimes adding a little extra, such as, "I love you, my friend," but always with that same sincere, deliberate tone. I grew accustomed to hearing this. I even looked forward to hearing it, but I never really grew comfortable with it. After he said "I love you," I would always silently lower the headset into its cradle.

One night I went to a recovery meeting downtown and, following Roger's suggestions, struck up a conversation with a man after the meeting. He was pleasant, but clearly he seemed in better shape than me emotionally and intellectually. He had not required inpatient treatment and had managed to hang onto his job and apartment. I felt intimidated.

He invited me to dinner later that week.

I felt uncomfortable but accepted. On the subway home, I reminded myself that I was making progress. Roger had told me that feeling a little uncomfortable wasn't always a bad thing. This unfamiliar feeling I was experiencing must be what it feels like to become a little more socially adept.

On the appointed night, I showed up at my new friend's apartment. He rang me in to the delicious smells of roasting meat. I thought we were going out to a diner, so I was mildly surprised.

"Pork chops, vegetable, and garden salad," he said. He wore an apron and smiled confidently.

He shooed me into the living room and finished in the kitchen. There were framed prints on the walls and everything looked tidy. I thought about the bare walls in my room in the Bronx, the mattress flopped on the floor. I reminded myself that feeling a little uncomfortable wasn't always a bad thing. I was starting over.

When we were finally seated at the dining room table, I picked a spring of parsley from the roast pork in front of me. I didn't know what to say. Even my mother didn't put little sprigs of parsley on my dinner.

My friend cleared his throat and said, "When I first discovered I was a homosexual. . ."

I kept my face composed, but when I heard the word, "homosexual," I felt alarmed. "You're gay," I interrupted.

My friend nodded cheerfully and continued his story.

My mind raced. The context of the entire evening shifted. I was suddenly in a weirdly familiar place, but the circumstances were unlike anything I had ever experienced before. I had always carefully orchestrated encounters with gay men, but this evening was all improvisation. I tried to recall the context of our previous conversations to see if I could get a handle on my feelings, but it was too hard to sort out. Had I been too solicitous? Was I giving off a gay vibe?

And then this dark thought: If he was gay, then what did that make me? *Was I his date?* Was I obligated to have sex with him?

For free!

What if I didn't like dinner?

The food smelled really good and I was hungry. I considered my options: I could just make a break for the door and race into the street, but that would clearly be overreacting. My friend stopped talking and soon he stopped eating, too. He looked at me with a flat expression.

"We don't have to do anything. . ." he paused, ". . . *sexual*."

I laughed nervously.

I picked up the flatware and started sawing up the meat and forking it into my mouth. I gulped ice water from the glass at my elbow. I even powered through the salad. The food was delicious. Halfway through the meal, it became obvious to both me and my friend that I was going to eat and run.

He sat with his arms folded, his dinner growing cold in his plate. "You might as well get used to it," he said, curtly. "You're in Manhattan now—all the men here are gay!"

On the train ride home, I felt humiliated.

I was angry with myself for acting so naïve. I was angry with Roger for asking me to ignore my uncomfortable feelings and for having me shake hands with the people to my right and to my left. But mostly I was angry that I continued to remain without a friend, despite having pushed myself the past few weeks.

When I got to the apartment, it was past 10:00 p.m. I called Roger anyhow. I thought I had cooled off, but as I explained what happened, I almost cried. I was shocked at the depth and intensity of my feelings.

"He shouldn't have done that," Roger said.

I felt grateful for Roger taking my back. I settled down and listened to the syrupy cadence of his voice. He said it was a given that people in the program would occasionally give you bad advice, treat you rudely, and sometimes hit on you, even if you were new.

Despite all of that, he insisted the program still worked.

I found listening to Roger almost like taking narcotics. He seemed so certain of himself, his priorities. I would occasionally chirp, "How so?" or something similar to keep him talking. Otherwise, I would just allow his voice to lull me into a quiet, calm place.

"The program isn't about getting good advice or being treated kindly, although you may very well find all of that. The program is about the steps. Every day you refrain from drugs and alcohol—whether you realize it or not—you work one or more of the steps."

"The program works," Roger said. "You can trust it."

Next morning, I found Mickey in the kitchen. I told him about being invited to dinner the night before by a guy from the recovery meeting.

"You know what he told me?" I asked, hoping to shock Mickey.

"Said he was half-a-fag?" Mickey was fussing with eggs in the fry pan and didn't look up.

I gasped, genuinely surprised. "How did you know?"

Mickey snorted.

He said something about being twice my age, shook his head and smiled. I was growing tired of always feeling like such a bumpkin, but I was grateful to be back in Mickey's good graces.

A friend from Rockford had given me a lead on a job with a non-union construction crew. Mickey got this information and passed it on to me. The job was a laborer position that paid about the same as the plant job.

Any job seemed better than the one I had. I eagerly applied.

* * *

"Blood clot, man," Damon said. "*Bloooood clot.*"

Damon was a middle-aged Jamaican, with a large belly and a bald head. He was sitting on an upturned bucket of drywall compound, eating his lunch. He wore a soiled T-shirt and paint-stained jeans, like everyone else on the five-man crew.

"Blood clot" was Damon's favorite phrase. He used it to express everything from surprise and indignation, to scorn or even threats of physical violence. Between bites of an oversized sandwich, he told a bawdy story about a request for sex his wife had made the previous night. His accent was so thick I only caught snatches of his story, but even so I was amused. The rest of the crew listened and laughed. It was Friday afternoon and we were working at an old estate somewhere north of the Bronx, in a neighborhood of large, expensive properties.

This was my fourth week on the job. I had been on enough labor crews in the past to know I wasn't going to work out on this one. I hustled to clean up messes or carry heavy loads, but the bigger problem was that I had no real trade skills, and couldn't find my place as part of the crew. To bond with a group of men like this wasn't terribly difficult, but I couldn't seem to find a firm footing anywhere and made zero progress.

The few attempts I made at fitting in were uncomfortable. On Fridays, they brought coolers filled with beer to the job, took a late lunch, and drank and told stories before leaving early for the weekend. My first Friday on the job, the crew chief, a stocky man who spoke with a thick Boston accent grew alarmed when the cooler was set down next to me.

"Don't put the cooler next to that guy!" the crew chief said.

I looked up in surprise. Another man reached into the cooler and drew out a cold bottle of beer. The crew apparently knew I had been in treatment.

The crew chief shrugged sheepishly and reached for his own bottle of beer. "Is this going to be okay?"

"Beer?" I said. "S' cool." I tried to make a joke to lighten the mood. "If anyone is going to tie off and shoot heroin, that might be a problem."

I grinned.

The crew chief raised his eyebrows. "You shot heroin?" he asked. From the other side of the room I heard Damon emit a low, plaintive moan: "Blooooooood clot."

*   *   *

Working on the construction crew felt like riding a slow-moving train into a brick wall. After work, I would duck into a recovery meeting in Hell's Kitchen or near Grand Central before riding the train home. These meetings were filled with New York's working class Irish, Italians, and Latinos, and the spiritual talk had a strong Christian flavor with much talk about the power of prayer. People in this meeting were fond of saying that to be successful in recovery you had to get down on your knees in the morning, and then get down on your knees again at night.

I found the phrase "Get down on your knees" to be an odd euphemism for prayer and had to restrain myself from snickering. Whenever I heard it, my mind always seemed to go to a lewd place. I heard it so often, I imagined it was a program-wide saying, like "One Day at a Time" or "But for the Grace of God." I was torn between my desire to stay in recovery and my cynicism about prayer. In the face of soon having to search for another job, I decided to try anything, even morning and evening prayer.

I got Roger on the phone and told him about this decision. I said, "I am getting down on my knees in the morning, and I am getting down on my knees again at night. Does that seem about right to you?"

There was an uncomfortable silence.

I felt my face grow hot. I wished I had not used the euphemism I had heard in the ethnic Midtown meetings.

Finally Roger said, "Are we talking prayer?"

"*Yes*," I said, trying to hide my irritation. Every time I thought I had my finger on the pulse of how I ought to act, I seemed to miss by a wide mark.

"I think you should pray constantly," he said. "Every waking minute that your mind is not actively engaged in something, you should pray."

"Holy shit," I snorted. "Really?"

I assumed he meant that I was so damaged that I needed more prayer than even the Italians, the Irish, or any of the other hard-bitten New Yorkers in the Midtown meetings. But then he went on to describe his outlook on prayer, and I realized it had little to do with me.

"When Martin Luther King talks about going to the mountain top," Roger said, "nobody thinks he put on his hiking boots. We understand he is speaking metaphorically. This is why you pray. You want to train yourself to look at the world metaphorically—as if you were looking at the world through a spiritual lens. Prayer is like exercise. You pray to exercise your spiritual muscles."

I had never heard anything like this in the meetings. It worked to ease my cynicism about prayer, if not my skepticism about my chances of staying in recovery. Roger asked how my new job was going. I admitted things were working out poorly. I hated it. He suggested looking for something I liked.

As always, he reminded me to pay attention to my feelings.

And then he added, "And pray."

* * *

Almost two eventful years after I'd gotten off the Greyhound bus in Times Square to start my recovery, I walked onto the campus of Bronx Community College.

Although it was early December, the sun sparkled in the sky. A brisk wind blew across campus. I felt nervous and excited, like the feeling you get going into a department store to shoplift, or when you hit a working vein and see that first little rosebud of blood in the barrel of a syringe.

One corner of the grounds held a few old buildings, with domed roofs and row upon row of tall wood-silled windows. Most of the other buildings were nondescript and newer—concrete block affairs with fold-out aluminum windows. Grand old trees bordered a wide, cracked pavement that circled a grassy courtyard. Various half-finished construction projects were cordoned off with yellow warning tape. Fall had gone out wet, leaving huge puddles of mud dotting the grounds. I had to step over a mud-spattered traffic barrier that lay on its side, yellow warning light blinking merrily into the dirt. Things were just broken down enough that I didn't feel too overwhelmed by that fact that I was on a college campus, attempting to sign up for classes. A small group of students pointed me toward the administrative offices.

In my plaster-stained work jeans, I sat at a desk and took a battery of placement exams in a starkly fluorescent-lit classroom. There were a dozen other students who all looked as if they had just gotten off work, too.

Two weeks later I got a slip of paper in the mail that said I required remedial math and remedial English classes. When I mentioned this to Roger, he said optimistically that I had to start somewhere, but I already felt upbeat and even the idea of needing remediation couldn't get me down. Roger had been reminding me to pay attention to my feelings so often that I had now zeroed in on this one key fact: this was the first thing I had been involved with in New York that clearly felt like a win in every direction. College would not fire me. College would not stop sleeping with me. College wouldn't scold me for not cleaning the apartment. The only real problem was finding the money for tuition in time for the next semester, which started in a few weeks. When I mentioned this to Roger, he said he would give me the tuition as a gift—about three hundred dollars.

I told him I couldn't take his money, but he insisted. He said he could afford it. I knew I needed to be in that classroom and didn't put up much of a fight.

A few weeks earlier, before Thanksgiving, the crew chief had approached me at the job site when I was alone, chipping paint in a back room. He said the company was doing poorly and would have to cut back. He was soft-spoken and sounded apologetic.

He said, "What do you need from this job?"

I had no idea what he meant. I told him as much and he repeated himself.

He must have been asking me to negotiate a severance package, but I had never been given anything more than a kick in the pants at the end of employment, so I negotiated poorly. I said that if I could keep the job through the holidays, I would be okay.

I felt ashamed that I was losing my job. I didn't mention the conversation to Roger or Mickey. I walked around with a lump in my chest through the month of December, hoping for a miracle. When the first of the year came, I got my final paycheck.

When I finally broke the news to Mickey, he took it badly. We were still going to outpatient aftercare groups at Rockford. People from our peer group were relapsing at a high rate. The relapses seemed to follow a predictable pattern. One of the warning signs included an inability to hold a job. Of course, the person who was relapsing always had an excellent rationale for why the jobs were lost. I wondered if I were just deluding myself as I explained the reasons for the loss of my job to the rest of the group.

Alone in our apartment after a particularly contentious group meeting at Rockford, Mickey asked, "Don't you care about anything?"

Having just started classes, I shot back, "I care about school."

Fortunately for me, this was the truth.

* * *

I enjoyed school immensely.

My remedial math teacher was a slender West Indian man with long, slim fingers. He had such a thick accent I could never be sure if I was confused by the algebra he taught or the way he expressed himself. I asked him to repeat himself a lot and he did so with good cheer. English was taught by an uninspired older woman. I shamed myself early in the semester by exclaiming, "A subject and a verb in *every* sentence?" The ripple of laughter reminded me of high school, where I was the kid always quick to make a joke. But I hadn't intended to make everyone laugh this time. I had been reacting more or less instinctively to the anxiety of being in a classroom filled with strangers.

The teacher looked at me and smiled wanly with tired eyes. I felt small, but I resolved to do better. Later in the semester, the teacher read an essay out loud to the class as a good example of a persuasive essay. As she began to read, I realized the words were mine. Using one of the prescribed topics, I'd made a passionate argument for leniency toward juvenile offenders. I kept my eyes on the desktop in front of me, but I felt a warm pleasure grow in my cheeks and a grin I couldn't suppress.

I took evening classes, so my days were free to look for work. I only had enough money in the bank for a week or two of living expenses at a time. Friends from meetings invited me to do odd jobs for money, and sometimes they invited me to stay for dinner. I always accepted, but it left me feeling like a burden to these people I hardly knew. I did the jobs the best I could, ate the food placed in front of me, and pocketed the money slipped into my hand before I went home.

Using the school bulletin board, I found a job opening at a pizza parlor in uptown Manhattan, just south of Harlem. The owner was a dark-haired Albanian, about my age, who had in his employ only two types of workers:

cooks who spoke Albanian and delivery guys who spoke Spanish. He needed someone who spoke English to answer the phones and run the register, especially during the brisk evening business on weekends, when the students from Columbia University kept the ovens hot and the register chiming.

He hired me.

My first night on the job I offered an exemplary performance.

There were three phones near the register and they would all clamor at once. I would pick up, greet and ask the caller to hold, and then repeat this until all the phones were off their hooks. At that point, I returned to the first caller and got his or her order and address. In between calls, I rang up retail orders or drew cold drinks from the soda fountain. After a few hours of this it was time for the Albanian Pizza King to lock the glass doors; the evening was over.

In his tiny basement office, I asked the Pizza King exactly how much the job paid, reminding him that the bulletin board notice had suggested a rate between seven and ten dollars an hour. He seemed to be in a good mood and asked aloud how much he should pay me. I suppose he meant it as a rhetorical question, but I quickly answered, "You're asking me? I say ten. Ten dollars an hour."

There was an uncomfortable silence.

I tried my best to smooth it over by smiling cheerfully. I knew better than to say anything more. My proposal hung in the dank basement air between us.

"Okay," the Pizza King said, after a moment. "Ten."

He didn't sound quite so cheerful.

For ten dollars an hour, the Albanian Pizza King expected a lot from me, and I tried my best to deliver. He paid me in cash, so I was earning more than ever before. Soon he left me to run the shop on my own, spending his evenings down in the basement. Or, after slipping on his shades and combing his dark hair back, he might duck out of the shop for a few hours in the early evening.

One night I took a call from an old woman who asked how many slices there were in a large pie. "Twelve," I said, just as all the other phones started to ring. I asked her to hold and did my little act with the phones. When I got her back on the line, she asked for three plain, two pepperoni, four mushroom, and three sausage.

It seemed like a lot of pizza. I asked if she were having a party and she said they were. I took her address and wrote the order up: a dozen large pies.

When the Spanish-speaking delivery guy saw the order, he balked. He scrutinized the address with the Pizza King. Sometimes fake orders came in to lure delivery personnel into an ambush. I assured them there was no need to worry; it was an old woman having a party. The Pizza King nodded his head but recommended caution. Delivery was a cash business and there was always the risk of robbery.

Ten minutes after the order went out, a call came in on the Pizza King's private line. He took the call and spoke in Spanish. Rubbing his chin, he glared at me.

After he hung up, the Pizza King stood by me at the register. He said quietly, "You know that order? She didn't want twelve pizzas. She wanted one large pie with twelve different slices. We sent her almost two hundred dollars' worth of pizza."

I groaned.

He reached into his pocket and took out a roll of cash. He peeled off a hundred dollars in twenties. "Here," he said. "I can't use you anymore."

I apologized, but the Albanian Pizza King just grunted. His lips were a tight little line across his face.

I didn't want to take his money, but it didn't seem wise to turn it down either. Stuffing the cash in my pocket, I took off my apron, and headed for the door.

I felt terrible as I walked to the train. To get home, I had to ride downtown, take a crosstown train, then another train back uptown. Rocking back and forth on the slow-moving local train, I had a lot of time to think about what had happened.

I kept reviewing in my mind the conversation I'd had with that old woman. I saw how the mistake had been made, but I didn't see any good way that I could have avoided it. In the meetings, the whole idea is that if you do your part, then God does His part. Together—you and God—were supposed to find a way into recovery.

What had been my part? I reviewed all of the decisions I had made since I entered recovery. I had come to New York to avoid getting sent to jail. Good decision. After the Pennsylvania judge pardoned me, I returned to New York. Then I realized it was foolish to return to Pennsylvania and stayed in New York. Two more good decisions. I started attending recovery meetings for alcoholics because I discovered the counselors at Rockford drank and it pissed me off. Now I was attending meetings on my own, calling my sponsor, and even praying. Good decisions all, and I didn't see how I could have made better ones.

My part also seemed to be finding and applying for work. Certainly my part included showing up for work, even if the only people who spoke English were the customers and an Albanian King of Pizza. My part arguably also included using sign language to communicate with my colleagues (thumbs up on that delivery, amigo; or a wave, a point of a finger, or rub of my tummy for the cook). All of this seemed to be my part.

I didn't see how my part included the intangibles, the stuff you couldn't possibly see coming, like wacky little old ladies holding pizza parties on Amsterdam Avenue.

The train stopped, its pneumatic doors opened. Like a commercial I'd seen too many times, in shuffled Chopper Cassidy. This time, he wore dark Wayfarers. His jeans were torn and stained. I didn't even bother to catalogue our differences.

"Somebody," I spoke slowly and clearly to the empty train car, "is not doing their part."

Chopper Cassidy flopped into a seat and the train lurched forward. He looked tired and pale. He didn't look at me.

"Not going to mention any names here," I said. "But I think it's fairly obvious to the casual observer that *someone*—name begins with a G and ends with a D—might be falling down on the job."

Chopper Cassidy had nothing to say to that one. He, too, seemed defeated, letting his body sag with the movement of the train.

I laughed harshly and sunk my head in my hands. I would call Roger tomorrow and listen to his interpretation of all this. I couldn't imagine what he could say that would make me feel better, but I believed he'd think of something.

And, for now, that was enough.

I sat like that, with my head in my hands, until I heard my stop called on the train's loudspeaker. When I looked up, Chopper Cassidy was gone.

*　*　*

Roger quietly listened to me explain about how I lost the pizza job.

I had gone through the story with Mickey the night before. Each time I described how it happened, I came to understand it a little better. The pounding shame I felt over losing the job was beginning to pass, and I began to see my mistake for what it was—unfortunate circumstance.

I expected Roger to confirm this, or to comfort me in some way. I expected him to say something about my Higher Power, or how I was going to be taken care of.

Instead he said, "Well—you won't starve."

His voice sounded grave. I felt myself grow anxious.

I started talking faster. I pointed out the spiritual distribution of labor stuff I had been thinking about on the train ride home. "My part," I said, "is to start looking for work again on Monday." I suggested that maybe my Higher Power had an even better job waiting for me.

Roger said he thought I was right.

But again I thought I heard a note of concern in his voice. In some small hidden part of my soul, I felt terrified to hear that concern, but I didn't dare ask him about it. If he really were feeling apprehensive, I certainly didn't want to know. I assured him that come Monday morning, I would head over to campus and look for work again.

I hung up with Roger and had an uneventful Sunday afternoon.

When I felt myself grow anxious, I reminded myself that all I could do was my part. If everything else went to hell, that part wasn't up to me (I wasn't going to mention any names here).

I came up with a list of things I could do to influence my success:

I could go to a meeting.

I could raise my hand and speak at the next meeting.

I could get some rest.

The litany of tasks small and great was literally endless. All things I could do to ensure my success. I suddenly felt powerful.

Later that evening just as the sun had dipped below the horizon, while the sky was still a deep violet, the phone rang. I padded into the hall to answer. The Pizza King asked if I wanted to work. I was too shocked to respond right away. I could hear the crowd in the pizza shop. Someone was clamoring for a refill of fountain soda.

"Come on. I need you. You wanna work or not?"

I thought about having been fired. I thought about my plans to look for work at the school the next morning. I thought about my Higher Power's plans for me to get a new job, possibly an even better job than this one. I thought about all these things in the space of a few short seconds, then I found my voice.

"Yes." I said. "I want to work."

He told me to get down there as quick as possible and then he hung up.

I laughed out loud.

I reached for the phone to call Roger and tell him the great news. As I started to dial his number, I stopped. I realized I could tell Roger tomorrow— my part probably involved getting my ass into Manhattan as fast as I could tonight.

CHAPTER 4

COURAGE

I stood at the back of the narrow bursar's office, building up enough nerve to approach the counter and discuss my financial circumstances in order to apply for financial aid. There were three or four people behind the counter and a few more on my side of the counter. I was there to ask if I was entitled to financial aid, and how the school decided such things. Determining my eligibility seemed crucial to getting anywhere with college. However, I was loathe to share my situation with total strangers, especially the young students working behind the counter.

"Can I help you?" A thin, dark-haired student with a wispy mustache turned to me. I grinned, my knee-jerk response to feeling intimidated.

To ease us into the conversation, I announced that I knew next to nothing about financial aid and asked for a quick primer on how to apply.

The student rolled his eyes and sighed.

He flopped a sheaf of forms in front of me and began racing through the requirements. I instantly regretted having taken the clueless approach with him. I had actually reviewed and even started filling out the financial aid forms, so I wasn't completely in the dark. I'd found out that because I had lived in the Bronx during treatment, I was now eligible for the cheaper rate for New York City residents. But there were certain eligibility issues about which I could find no information. Would the fact that I had been on welfare—huge implications for child support—during my stay at Rockford hamper my eligibility for financial aid?

I felt ashamed that I had been on assistance and—even worse—that I had attended inpatient drug treatment. I wanted to get my eligibility questions answered without revealing too much personal information. I also wanted to understand the system better to see how much I could count on financial aid for the upcoming semesters or if I needed to come up with a different strategy to pay for college.

The thin young man with the mustache slipped into a dismissive tone, and I realized he probably wasn't going to be much help to me at all. He was rattling off a list of things I'd need to address before he could answer any of my questions. One of his requirements caught me off guard: "You're going to need both your parents' tax returns for the past five years."

"Wait, what?" I balked.

He raised his brow imperiously.

"My dad is dead," I said.

I immediately felt foolish for trotting out the death of my father from ten years prior, but I couldn't imagine attempting to explain my complicated family situation to this student. The young man looked at me with a bland expression.

To rescue the conversation, I chuckled and said, "And I really don't even speak to my mother."

He let this information sink in for a moment. Then he nodded curtly and said, "You're just going to have to make up with her."

He launched into more things he might need from me, but I had already stopped listening. I felt embarrassed and irritated that he had correctly surmised my poor relationship with my mother. But the thought of asking Mom for her tax records filled me with dread. I had a long history of rattling off convincing stories about needing this check or that document signed—every story uniquely compelling—but each ultimately leading to the same dark place: Mom a little poorer, a little more guarded. This request would have been for a legitimate need, but it didn't really matter; anything that required an impassioned plea to Mom from me just wouldn't work. I couldn't do it. This was a deal breaker. My ability to finance school seemed to rest on this decision. I raised my hand to interrupt like an elementary school student.

"Why do we need the tax records?" I asked.

He pursed his lips and exhaled noisily.

I felt terrible for bringing us back around to this same point, but I wanted to understand the matter better, especially if it were going to upend my chances for aid. He dismissed my question, but I interrupted and asked him again. He looked at me incredulously and started complaining about his circumstances. He said he had almost completed his degree, but that the best job he could find was helping students like me fill out simple forms.

We went on like this for a few minutes—him growing openly more hostile, and me stubbornly asking for more information—until finally he ended it by asserting that he had explained financial aid as well as could be humanly expected. As he said, "humanly expected," he tossed a pencil onto a nearby table and it bounced noisily in the eerie quiet of the room. All eyes in the room seemed to be on us. I kept my own eyes on the counter.

A young woman approached the young man helping me, and she put her hand on his bicep. In a gentle voice, she suggested he take a break and offered to finish with me. With a disgusted sigh, he retreated, leaving me with the young woman, who seemed kind and eager to help. Taking up the forms in her hand, she started to interview me. One of the first questions she asked was if I had ever been in an institution before.

My mouth dried up.

She was eye-catching, with her long hair parted in the middle, and a young, inquisitive face. I was loath to list all the time I had spent in various rehabs—not to mention the few weeks in Dauphin County Prison, the aborted stay in a hospital detox, or even the brief spell at the homeless shelter here in New York. There was a beat of silence as I considered my options. I looked around the room and licked my lips.

"Do you mean *learning* institutions?" I finally asked.

"Yes," she said.

I let out an audible sigh.

"No," I laughed. "First time."

There was an awkward pause and she looked at me curiously.

I figured things couldn't get much worse, so I quickly blurted out the question about welfare. To save face, I presented it rhetorically—"Say someone had recently been on welfare and wanted financial aid," I asked. The girl said she didn't think it mattered. She mentioned that no one had ever asked her such a question before. She asked another woman—an older, matronly looking woman with sturdy legs—who immediately dismissed the idea as irrelevant, barely looking up from the tall stack of forms she was sorting. I found this comforting.

As we continued to work our way through the form, I circled back to the issue of my mother's tax forms and discovered the underlying issue was whether my mother had claimed me as a tax deduction. I triumphantly announced that I had been filing my own taxes for years.

And just like that, I had done all I could to apply for financial aid.

* * *

Mickey moved out.

He had found a smaller apartment where he could live with his girlfriend. When he first announced his intentions, I felt abandoned and sulked, mostly knowing that my behavior was irrational, but feeling incapable of any other response. With Roger's help, I eventually conceded the inevitability of Mickey's move and my own inability to change it. With Mickey's help, I found a smaller apartment where I could live alone. Although the new apartment was less expensive than the Pelham Parkway apartment, my total monthly expenses had risen and my income wasn't enough to cover the new apartment.

Through a college work-study program, I found temporary work at the administrative offices of CUNY, the City University of New York, on the Upper East Side of Manhattan. I worked for full-time staff and faculty members and with other work-study students. Our tasks included filing, and occasionally answering phones, but a lot of the time there was nothing to do, so we just hung out and looked busy. The days were mind-numbingly dull, but the evening classes were challenging and made it all seem worthwhile. Plus, I was making ends meet.

Most of the furniture and appliances in my old apartment had been Mickey's, so the new place felt bare and desolate. A previous tenant had left a laminated table in the kitchen where I spent most of my time doing class work—pale yellow walls and the hum of an empty refrigerator. One room held my mattress and a few stacks of clothes, and another room held nothing at all—cold brown linoleum tiles and textured walls. At night, the naked windows let in great rectangles of street light that gave the walls a fluorescent glow.

I tried to find more work, but my all-too-familiar lack of confidence and growing sense of impending calamity made it hard to apply, much less interview. The work-study job was coming to an end. We had been told that some work-study students were occasionally transitioned to permanent positions, but there was no indication of how or when this would happen, or if it had ever even happened in the past. At some point that summer, I began to feel a great weight on my chest, and I stopped leaving my apartment, except for school. Roger cajoled and encouraged me to keep looking for jobs. What he said made perfect sense, but I couldn't bring myself to do it.

One day I just stopped going to work.

After a few days, Tanisha, one my fellow work-study students called and asked me if I was planning on coming back to work again. I liked this girl and often walked her to the uptown train after work. She was a single mother about my age—creamy skin and delicate hairs on her shins that she refused to shave, which made her seem all the more earthy and wild. To pass the time, we liked to talk about our kids. I hadn't told her my whole story, but she knew I needed work, had few job skills, and no family nearby.

I told her I had given up on finding work at the college.

"Dean Bernstein wants to hire you," Tanisha said. She was whispering into the phone. I felt certain she was lying but it pleased me to hear the concern in her voice.

"Bullshit," I laughed. "He does not."

"No, really," Tanisha whispered. "Dean Bernstein wants to talk to you."

"Why are you whispering?"

"I can't get into that right now," she said.

She asked if I would to talk to the dean myself.

Dean Bernstein was a towering man with fine white hair and a booming voice. He had an impressive title but as far as I could tell, he commanded the entire floor by virtue of his personality. One time I'd been working in the office and he stormed in, slammed the newspaper down onto his secretary's desk, and asked her to phone one of the deans from SUNY, the State University of New York. He said it was an urgent matter and kept asking for updates throughout the morning. When he finally got his man on the phone, Dean Bernstein took the call at his assistant's desk in the large common room. He loudly proclaimed that "Dart Man," a minor thug who had been in the headlines the entire summer—his name given him by the tabloids for using a blow gun to skewer the buttocks of attractive young women riding the subway—had been a graduate of the SUNY system. The whole office stopped to watch Dean Bernstein, who took the call, grinning ear-to-ear, one fist on his hip. *What are you teaching our young men up there, the future leaders of our fair state?* The SUNY dean called foul because the information had come from one of the tabloids. But Dean Bernstein protested, even as his secretary hurriedly found a corroborating story in the *New York Times*. After he hung up, grinning and triumphant, Dean Bernstein pointed out to all of us watching him, that this same SUNY dean made similar calls to him every time a CUNY graduate was arrested, which made this particular victory sweet indeed. Dean Bernstein clapped his hands together and cackled, making a good-natured sound.

I felt intimidated by the bigness of his personality that lonely afternoon, but I wanted to call Tanisha's bluff, or at least keep her on the phone for a few more minutes. She asked me to hold, and I waited for at least fifteen or twenty minutes. Every so often Tanisha would come back on the line, whisper that it would just be another few seconds, or she might just hiss, *Wait, wait.*

I eventually realized she might not be bluffing and grew anxious. I didn't want to appear weak, so I stayed on the line, determined to call the whole thing off at the first opportunity. But the next time she picked up, she said, "Hold for Dean Bernstein," in that sing-song voice receptionists always seem to use.

I felt a ripple of panic.

Next thing I knew, Dean Bernstein was on the phone.

I stuttered something inarticulate and lame. Dean Bernstein listened for a few seconds, and then took over the conversation. I was happy to let him lead. He reiterated the same thing we had been told all summer long—if there were a need come fall, then some of the work-study students might get jobs. But, he added pointedly, you had to actually show up to get the job. I felt indicted and ashamed. Even I didn't understand why I had stopped coming to work, so it seemed hopeless to try to explain. I stuttered something else—a diplomatic retreat—and then said I'd be in the next day. As we said our goodbyes, I suddenly felt a surge of gratitude—as if I had just been rescued from some terrible fate—and I thanked Dean Bernstein for calling me.

"I didn't call you," he said. "You called me."

There was an uncomfortable silence.

"Exactly," I said. "Thank you."

Nothing had changed, but somehow everything had changed. I felt so touched that Tanisha had called me and then orchestrated getting Dean Bernstein on the phone.

I went back to work the next day. In the fall, I got a permanent part-time job and kept it for most of the remainder of my time in New York. After that summer, I never saw Tanisha again. In the few weeks before she left, I never asked her what she had said to get Dean Bernstein on the phone. I thought of it, but we never spoke of it. I wasn't ready to admit what a coward I had been, depressed and waiting in my empty apartment to see what would happen next. For her, I like to think that it was all about improvisation, just a virtuoso single parent playing it by ear, seeing what she could do to make some small change in the world.

* * *

I followed Joey up Swatara Street. He was still just a noodle of a boy, all sun-browned arms and skinned knees. We were trekking up the high school hill to pass a baseball—me carrying his stepdad's glove, him loping three paces ahead. I hadn't lived on this block in years and didn't recognize many of the neighbors who sat out on their front porches. Joey knew everyone. He waved at some people across the street, then shouted to someone else sitting on a porch.

Sometimes he would stop, address someone on their porch. "My dad's home," he'd say. "He lives in New York."

I'd nod, smile.

I felt vaguely uncomfortable meeting so many people, wondering how much they knew of my story, or if they knew anything at all. On these weekend visits, I tried to let Joey take charge. I followed him. We did whatever he wanted to do, as long as it didn't cost too much.

We were halfway up the hill and it dawned on me how difficult it would be for me to reach out—wave, or just say hello—to that many people. "You're popular, son," I said. "People really like you."

Joey stopped. I wasn't expecting him to do that, and I strode past him and then looked over my shoulder to see what had caused him to pull up short. He was standing there with his mouth open.

"Me?" he asked.

"You didn't know that?" I laughed. "You're very outgoing. You know everyone, everyone knows you."

His eyes welled up with emotion, and then he blushed—bright red strawberries across both his cheeks. I was surprised—as much by his reaction as by my ability to elicit it with such small praise.

He put his head down and started walking with me.

"I wasn't like that when I was little," I said. "I'm not even like that now, but I wish I were." I didn't want to overplay it or embarrass him, but I knew I'd said the right thing.

He needed my perspective. And I wanted to give it to him.

* * *

Permanent part-time employment at CUNY required paperwork.

I had to go to the business offices on the second floor of my building to fill out forms. The second floor was staffed by clerks and typists, mostly middle-aged and older, a few attending night classes, but none of the academics—graduate students or Ph.D.s—from the fourth floor where I worked. As I filled out my paperwork, I noticed one of the male clerks—a younger man—staring at me with open curiosity. He was neatly shaved and dressed like most of the other clerks, in button down shirts and slacks. Some even wore ties. I felt awkward in my combat boots, jeans and long, unruly hair that could never be counted on to stay flat.

I learned I would need to be photographed, so I ducked into the bathroom to do something with my hair. Using handfuls of sink water, I tamed it as best I could. As I waited for the woman to take my picture, the well-dressed young clerk who had been staring at me earlier came to stand next to me. He rubbed his chin and looked at my damp hair.

"Did you just put water in your hair?" he asked.

"I did," I murmured.

He shook his head. The woman operating the camera, a clerk in a floor-length dress, chuckled at our exchange. She shooed the other clerk away in Spanish, and then snapped my picture.

I liked the people up on my floor better.

On nice days, I would take my sack lunch and eat in a small park on the bank of the East River. A small mom-and-pop Irish delicatessen—Shannon's Deli—served the whole neighborhood. I would stop in for a can of soda to drink with my lunch.

On the way back to the office one day, I went into Shannon's Deli for cigarettes. In a burst of desperation, I asked if I could speak to the owner about a job. The old woman bristled that she was, in fact, Mrs. Shannon. She asked if I had ever worked retail and I told her about the pizza shop. I explained that I already worked part time at the CUNY building and was willing to load, unload, stock shelves—whatever. I imagined a weekend job. Possibly lifting things. She called for Dana, her daughter, a petite woman, with a no-nonsense disposition.

I repeated my pitch and tried to look cheerful. She asked if I could run a cash register and be in by 7:00 every morning.

I hated morning work.

"Morning?" I repeated weakly.

Dana grinned. "It's all we got."

The next morning I was on the sidewalk outside Shannon's at five minutes to seven. I tapped on the window and Mrs. Shannon tottered over and let me in. She showed me the register, gave me an apron, and told me to get ready for the morning rush. I tried to refuse the apron, but Mrs. Shannon insisted. I felt demeaned by wearing the apron—as if I had been demoted from office to retail clerk by donning this one accouterment.

I turned my back to the counter and tied on my apron. As I turned to face the rush, the delicatessen was filled with people—CUNY people. These were the early risers, the clerks from the second floor. I recognized some of them. They packed the store and stood in a line that snaked all the way back onto the sidewalk.

Someone started laughing. I felt my face heat up.

"You working here?" It was the smarmy clerk who had poked fun at my hair while I was getting photographed.

I breathed heavily and forced a smile.

"I am," I said.

"Did you lose your job?"

"No," I said. "I work here first, and then I work down there."

"You get me my coffee in the morning, and then you work down there?" He nodded toward the CUNY building, a doubtful look on his face.

I could see Mrs. Shannon didn't appreciate this exchange. I wasn't prepared for it either. It was one thing to serve anonymous customers, another to serve colleagues. I wondered if this arrangement would work out.

Mrs. Shannon snapped her fingers in the air over the counter.

"Come on, come on," she said. "We got a line here."

I got him his coffee and roll. Rang up his change. For the next hour and a half, I filled orders, drew coffee, and explained to the other CUNY clerks my presence behind the counter. There were a lot of grins. Some of the young guys would get bossy and bark out an order. Regular coffee was usually a dollop of cream and two sugars, but you always had to ask, because regular might mean double cream or four sugars to some folks. Early in the morning people were cranky and demanding about their coffee. Eventually there was a lull.

Mrs. Shannon said to take a little break, and we could expect another rush in half an hour. The next rush brought the professionals and academics from my floor and the chancellor's office. These people were more patient and there was less sarcasm, but I still had to explain my presence behind the counter. I had taken this job on a lark, not expecting it would demand so much from me socially. I wondered again at what I had gotten myself into. By mid-morning Dana showed up. Mrs. Shannon had a few words with Dana in the back, and then Dana came out grinning and even offered to make me a breakfast sandwich.

I had performed well.

I turned and found Dean Bernstein standing at the cash register. When he saw me, he did a double take and I quickly explained to him the new arrangement. With a shrug, I added that I needed the money, something I hadn't shared with anyone else, but felt that I needed to say to Dean Bernstein.

"Dana," he barked. "Ms. Dana Shannon, come out here."

Dana appeared from the back room.

"I understand you're raiding our workforce?" Dean Bernstein said in his mock stern voice, arms folded across his big chest.

I tried to hide my smile.

"You realize, of course, you're taking one of our finest young men?" He picked up his coffee and the paper sack with his buttered roll.

Dana grinned and apologized and then mugged with Dean Bernstein for a few more minutes.

"We're going to let it go this time," Dean Bernstein said, "but understand, Dana—we're drawing a line in the sand."

Winking to me, Dean Bernstein said, "See you in a bit."

I grinned back.

With Dean Bernstein on my side, I felt encouraged. A few minutes later Dana paid me in cash, and told me I was welcome to work the morning rush Monday through Friday. With part time jobs at Shannon's Deli and CUNY, I earned a living for the remainder of my time in New York City.

*   *   *

Before fall semester, I received mail from the financial aid office. I had qualified for aid, but it wasn't enough.

I called Roger. All summer he had been assuring me that if my Higher Power wanted me in college, I would find a way to pay for it. And if college wasn't for me, then something equally compelling would present itself. I didn't want to whine, but I didn't want something else. I wanted college.

We determined that there were two possible courses of action: apply for a government-backed loan or ask my family for help. The loan idea didn't seem too smart. I couldn't imagine anyone lending me that much money and even asking for such a lump sum felt a little dangerous. My Uncle Ward seemed like my best hope for getting family money, but this also seemed like a long shot. When my father died, my mother received his government pension, but Uncle Ward was made the beneficiary of Dad's life insurance policy. Dad had asked his brother to use the money to help me or my siblings go to college or meet other financial needs. Uncle Ward had already used some of this money on my behalf for a lawyer, a visit to rehab, and even bus fare to initially get me to New York City for this latest adventure. He took seriously his role as executor and didn't have much confidence in me or my recovery. I had asked him for money as recently as last spring and he had been curt, practically hanging up on me.

I explained all this to Roger, who said he thought I should ask my uncle again and offered some advice about how to proceed. "Your job," Roger said, "is to do all you can to get the money for school. That includes asking your uncle for help." I expressed how angry and adversarial my past conversations with my uncle had been. Clearly we would need a Plan B. Roger said that none of this mattered. He said my uncle's control over me getting into college was just an illusion.

"Your Higher Power is responsible for getting you into college," Roger said, "if college is the path you're supposed to follow." This was one of those things that Roger would say that sounded so corny and unlikely, but he would say it with so much conviction, that I'd feel a giddy little sense of joy lurking somewhere at the back of my mind. I wanted to believe we'd find a way to pay for college, but I knew my uncle much better than Roger did, so I began toying with the idea of applying for a loan.

Roger warned me not to get angry, to just ask for what I needed and then let go of the results. Before he hung up, Roger said that if I couldn't get my uncle to give me any money from the trust, to ask him to give me some of his own money instead.

I laughed.

"His own money?" I repeated incredulously.

"Sure," Roger said. "Tell him you really want to go to college, and so you're asking everyone you know for help."

We both laughed.

The next night I called my Uncle Ward. I slipped to the floor in my kitchen, hugged my knees to my chest, and traded some pleasantries.

Uncle Ward cut me off and asked what I wanted. I launched my pitch for money from the trust. He quickly shot me down, citing my previous withdrawals from the fund and the fact that he didn't trust me. He seemed to be itching for a fight. He launched into a speech on my lack of character, but I wasn't paying too close attention. My mouth dried up, and I waited for him to finish.

When he stopped talking, I said, "I hear you, Uncle Ward—how about you? Can you lend me the money?"

"I just told you no," he said.

"You said no about the trust," I said. "But I'm asking if *you* can lend me the money for school."

"Me?" he squeaked.

I choked back an urge to laugh and cleared my throat. "I'm asking everyone I know. I really want to go to college. If I can't use the trust, I'm probably going to need a loan."

There was utter silence on the other end of the phone for what seemed like an eternity. I had the good sense not to say anything, but just wait with the phone pressed to my sweaty ear.

Uncle Ward chuckled. "You sonofabitch—you're asking me for money? *Me?*"

"Yeah," I chuckled. "You're family, right?"

Uncle Ward laughed. Then he snorted. Then he sighed.

He told me he thought I had a lot of nerve. And then he said some other things I can't remember. Before we got off the phone, he said he'd consider giving me the money from the trust fund and asked me when classes started.

And this is how I paid for college: I called Uncle Ward at the start of each semester, explained how I was doing, and asked him to cut me another check for the next semester.

CHAPTER 5

INTEGRITY

I felt great.

I was holding two part-time jobs, maintaining an apartment, and getting ready to transfer to one of the senior colleges in the CUNY system. I hadn't seen Mickey or anyone else from Rockford in months, but I rarely felt lonely. I was going to recovery meetings two or three times a week, and had gotten a feel for how best to use the program to meet my needs.

In the past, attendance at recovery meetings had always made me feel crazy. I hated all the Johnny do-gooder advice and direction—much of it unsolicited and often contradictory. With Roger as my sponsor, I was learning how to stand up for myself with the people I met at meetings, but doing so diplomatically, without any hard feelings. This required confidence from me, which I was building, a little at a time, from providing for myself and going to school. Mostly this meant that I received criticisms or suggestions by saying things like, "I'll have to take a look at that." If someone was persistent and pointed with me, I might get them to back off by saying, "I'm starting to feel a little judged, here."

One day during the week when I had time off from work, I went to a mid-morning meeting across town and met Rose, a young woman who was new to recovery. Rose told me she had no job and complained of the many dull afternoon hours she had to fill. When the meeting ended, I invited her to my apartment for coffee. I knew this behavior was frowned upon, but my confidence was brimming. Most women would have ignored me. Some might have laughed or told me to fuck off. But Rose followed me home on the bus. She couldn't give me her phone number, so we met for afternoon trysts at the mid-morning crosstown meeting whenever I had time off work. I tried to be discreet about what we were doing but the old timers at the meeting caught on. They glared as we left the meeting. I tried to ignore them as best I could, but I started feeling guilty.

My confidence flagged. Finally I called Roger.

I sat on the floor of the kitchen in my apartment, the phone propped on my shoulder. I knew I could trust Roger, but I nervously worked my hands as I spoke.

He listened patiently, then he asked whether I thought this woman was capable of making good decisions so early in her recovery. I pointed out that Rose was an adult.

Roger asked if I felt as if I had been able to make good decisions early in my recovery. Good enough, I told him, offering as evidence my progress thus far.

Roger cut me off and this surprised me. His voice sounded exasperated, which pained me. "Do you have to do this?" he wanted to know.

I glanced around my empty apartment. What might I do instead? I couldn't afford to buy CDs or books. I rarely went to movies, just to avoid the risk of spending money on a bad one. Sex was one of the few pleasures that I could afford.

The guilt I felt earlier had somehow disappeared. I stopped playing nervously with my fingers and sat up straighter. The thought of the pain involved if I gave up this taboo pleasure outweighed the guilt I felt. And I was definitely feeling judged.

"Yes," I said. "I need to do this." I felt as confident as I sounded. The phone went silent for a beat, and I waited to hear what would come next.

"Okay then," Roger said. His voice had an even tone, a note of finality.

As soon as I heard that tone, my confidence crumbled. I felt awful.

I'd been prepared to fiercely advocate my position, but Roger was going to let me make my own decision. I sighed. Suddenly, my reasoning seemed poorly thought-out, based only on my own selfish needs. I felt deflated from bearing the responsibility for my own choices instead of distracting myself with an argument about principles.

I told Roger as much.

He chuckled.

He told me to relax. To see what happened next. He said he thought I was learning to spread my wings. In my past attempts at recovery, guys I had worked with would take on a wounded, "you'll-soon-rue-this-day" tone, but not Roger.

He seemed like one in a million.

* * *

After my shift, I raced from Shannon's Deli to the CUNY building. I had discovered that Hunter College, one of the senior colleges I was currently evaluating, had a small dormitory associated with it. The dorms weren't a secret, but they weren't common knowledge either. Hunter College's main campus was in Midtown Manhattan and the dorms were forty blocks south, near Bellevue.

As I was researching Hunter, I talked to a friend who was a student living in the dorm. She had wild, stringy brown hair and the body of an adolescent boy. She told me she got in by exaggerating a desperate situation with her family. "I told them my dad was abusing me," she said. She tilted her head down, looked me in the eye over her sunglasses, and then added, "*Sexually.*"

Pulling back, I grimaced. "Are you serious?" I asked.

"'Course not," she said, crushing out her cigarette with a matter-of-fact manner. "But they ate it up. That's how all the girls get a dorm room."

The rooms were inexpensive—less than half what I paid for rent in the Bronx—and because of this, prized. If I could get one, I could work less and attend classes more.

"Do you think I can get in?" I asked.

She looked me up and down, then sighed and punched her glasses higher on her nose. "I don't know," she said. "Tell them your dad is abusing you."

I wasn't going to lie about my situation, but I certainly didn't want to tell anyone the naked truth. I couldn't stop thinking about getting a room at the dorm. I wondered if I could find someone who would pull some strings for me.

As I thought more about it, I felt certain that Dean Bernstein was my one good hope. He was important, connected, and he liked me. If he couldn't help me, who could? I presented my case to him and he agreed. He hadn't known about the dorms, but he called one of his colleagues, Art, a research fellow and big baseball fan. Dean Bernstein said Art had spent a good bit of his teaching career at Hunter and would know who to ask.

Folding his arms across his chest, Art listened to my request. He glanced at Dean Bernstein, and then told us he would see what he could do.

* * *

The Friday night recovery meeting was close to my apartment, but worlds away from the mid-morning meetings on the other side of town. Held in a classroom of a small brick schoolhouse, my home group was a blue-collar discussion meeting with a working-class sensibility that reminded me of home. One night early that fall, we all got our coffee and then stuffed ourselves into the tiny desks that dotted the room.

I squeezed into a seat near my friend Richard.

Richard taught secondary school at one of the local public schools in the Bronx. We had been in recovery for about the same amount of time. He was a professional, about my age. We were in a room full of forty- or fifty-something laborers, short-order cooks, and firemen. One of the regulars was Archie, a red-faced Irishman with the features and discernment of a fireplug. He drove a gold, late-model Oldsmobile 88. He wore flannel shirts with the cuffs turned up to the elbow and always sat in the back of the meeting room. Each week, he said almost the exact same thing, no matter what the topic.

I had grown up around guys like Archie and was comfortable sipping coffee and cracking wise with him and the others, but I longed to be more like Richard who seemed so eloquent and insightful. Each time he spoke, he shaped whatever he had to say to conform to the topic at hand. Richard wasn't just making banal statements about feeling gratitude or blind acts of faith. He was exploring his day-to-day experience in a way few of the others seemed willing to try. He also had a wry sense of humor that I liked.

I often found myself trying to imitate Richard. I confided in him. I told him about my longing for a meaningful relationship with my son. At the meetings, I liked to talk about the things I was doing to promote the relationship, like wrestling a few minutes of long distance phone conversation out of him, or the jostling train visits to his home in Pennsylvania.

After one meeting broke up, Richard and I walked into the parking lot.

We stood watching Archie and the others chat or load themselves into their cars and drive off. I mentioned to Richard that I was evaluating the purchase of a portable CD player. The whole setup was about one hundred fifty dollars, plus the cost of CDs. I had found a small set of speakers with a built-in amplifier that I could use to listen to music at my apartment without the headphones. I could also use a CD player on the long train rides into work or Pennsylvania. Besides the phone, it would be the first appliance of any kind I had purchased since leaving treatment. The more I thought about lighting my apartment with music, the more eager I grew to have the means to do so. I was explaining the benefits of CDs over cassettes when I glanced over at Richard and noticed his frown.

"What?" I asked.

"Nothing." He looked away.

"What?" I insisted. Archie gunned his Olds to life and I had to squint from the sudden glare of his headlights. I held my hand up to shield my eyes, and the bright headlights cast a severe light on Richard's expression.

"Are you paying child support yet?" Richard asked. Turning his chin, he looked me right in the eye.

I dropped my hand and turned my head.

We both knew the answer. I often shared how Maryanne was after me to start paying child support. With the cost of school supplies and the apartment, I felt justified holding off on this obligation. Roger pointed out that Joey seemed well cared-for, even if I wasn't sending in the monthly checks.

"Maybe it's none of my business," Richard said.

"Maybe," I said.

* * *

I wiped the counter at Shannon's Deli, still mulling over the parking lot conversation from the previous Friday. This much was clear to me: my friend Richard was a prick. He was taking what I had said in meetings and using it against me. I felt bitter and disappointed. He was judging me. For days now, I had been trying to practice recovery principles—"Live and Let Live," "Let Go and Let God." I had even found myself praying for Richard's sorry ass, but nothing seemed to work. I wasn't making much headway.

Art walked up to the counter and smiled.

I stopped wiping and immediately assembled his order—regular coffee and a buttered roll—popped it into a brown paper bag, and then slid it toward him.

"On the house," I said, waving away his money.

"Thanks," Art nodded.

I grinned, placing my fists on the counter and leaning in toward him. "What can you tell me about the dorm room at Hunter?" I asked. "Any progress?"

Art sighed. He shook his head. "Have you ever considered moving back home with your parents?" he asked. "That's what most people do to get through college."

I snorted with disapproval and folded my arms. "Not an option," I said. "My family is in Pennsylvania."

"Take a train," Art said. "Commute."

"It's a four-hour trip," I said. "Fifty bucks one way."

"It doesn't cost $50," Art said.

"It doesn't?" I asked.

"I can get all the way to the other end of Long Island for much less than fifty bucks," Art said. He switched the brown paper bag from one hand to the other and licked his lips.

"My family isn't in Long Island," I said. "And besides, if I move out of state, my tuition goes up."

Art looked at me for a long moment and then he sighed.

"I'm sorry," he said. "Dorm rooms are tough. You can only get one if you fit the criteria for needing one. It's all very politicized. I've talked to everyone I know." He spread his arms. "I just can't help."

Running my hand across my forehead and back through my hair, I sighed. I pursed my lips and smiled and thanked him for trying. But I felt disappointed.

* * *

I called Roger from home.

I intended to tell him about the disappointing news I had received from Art. I wanted to hear him encourage me, to hear something cheerful about the Higher Power, or how everything would all work out in the end. Instead we started to discuss the conversation I'd had with Richard.

I felt pretty certain that Roger would agree with me that Richard's behavior was lacking. I imagined we would both acknowledge how inappropriate it was for him to have judged me, and then Roger and I would be free to move our conversation on to the business about the dorm. With the uncertainty about living at school, my anger with Richard had receded to mere background noise in my life. I was ready to "Let Go and Let God" as we said in the meetings. I had already purchased the portable CD player, which now rested on an upended plastic milk crate in my living room, a small monument to my increased earning power and newfound confidence. I could afford to be magnanimous.

I finished explaining about the CD player and Richard's comments.

Roger remained silent.

For a minute, I thought he hadn't been following the conversation. I was ready to jump back in and explain how I had already forgiven Richard for his rude behavior. By working the program, I no longer felt any anger or bitterness. If anything, I felt *sad* for him. I had seen this tactic employed in some of the upscale meetings in Manhattan, and I was eager to give it a try. I'm no longer mad, the hip urbanite might say, now I'm just sad. I was above Richard's judgmental superiority. He had transgressed, I would be forgiving.

I was really enjoying this business of working the program.

"If you wanted to start sending in your child support payments," Roger said, "you could go ahead and start sending them in."

"What!" I balked.

I had heard what he had said but was unable to grasp the direction the conversation had turned. "I thought you said Joey seemed well cared-for?"

My voice sounded more wounded than I intended.

"He does seem well cared-for," Roger said. "And if you don't think you can start sending the checks out just yet, then maybe you shouldn't. But if you think you can—well, there's nothing wrong with that either."

Roger started to go on, but I didn't catch much of whatever else he said.

I realized it was all back up to me again. Roger was going to support me whatever choice I made. Looking around the room, I glanced at the little CD player on its makeshift altar. I had to make a decision about child support. I wished I had someone more responsible than myself to rely upon.

*   *   *

My right leg bounced involuntarily as I sat in the chair. I let my eyes wander over all the stacks of books in the otherwise nondescript office of the administrator for the dormitory at Hunter College. He looked to be only a few years older than me. He sat in a chair at his desk and shuffled some paperwork. I started to explain to him about reducing my expenses. He folded his hands on the desk and waited for me to finish. I explained that my family lived in Pennsylvania and that I had been in New York for about three years. His eyes narrowed and he pursed his lips, but he remained silent. I knew it was time to come to the point, but a wave of nervous energy washed over me.

Finally I blurted, "I'm an addict."

He tilted his head. A curious half smile crept across his face. He had the look of a man waiting for the punch line of a joke.

My throat tightened and I felt my T-shirt stick to the small of my back. I stared at the top of the desk in front of me. "And an alcoholic," I added. "I came to New York City for a seat in a drug treatment facility." I explained to him about the homeless shelter, the Rockford facility, and the string of unsatisfying jobs. I told about discovering college at Bronx Community College.

After a few minutes, I risked looking up at his face.

His brow was furrowed. The smile on his face had disappeared.

I rushed to explain that I was working to rebuild ties with my family. I finished by announcing that I had a seven-year-old son and that I paid child support—which was true; I had sent a check to the New York City support enforcement office that very morning. I said that I thought if I could get a room at the dorm, I had a really good chance of getting a degree and building a future for myself.

I stopped talking. I could hear traffic from the street below. His phone rang and he pushed a button to make it stop.

"What kind of drugs?" he asked, pursing his lips.

"Heroin," I said softly.

He leaned back in his chair and the smile returned to his face.

I'd gotten a room at the dorm.

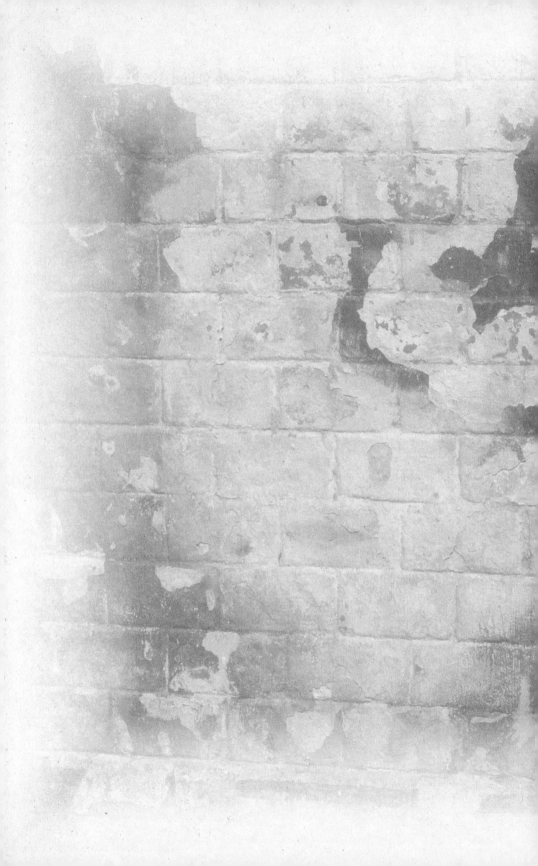

CHAPTER 6

WILLINGNESS

For non-custodial fathers, money is the root of all tension.

During telephone calls to Joey, Maryanne often took the line after we finished talking. "Did you send the check?" she'd want to know.

"It's in the mail," I'd tell her. And it was.

Although I kept up with child support, the amount was small, despite the additional money I sent to pay down the arrearage. Maryanne had not bothered me about support all through rehab and even for a while after I had finished. But once I started to pay, she quickly grew disillusioned with our arrangement.

"When are you going to get a real job?" she'd ask, exasperation lacing her voice.

These were the parts of the telephone calls where I had to be most careful. College *did* seem like a luxury. Sometimes it seemed like a huge reach for me to have organized so much of my life around getting a degree. None of my friends back home attended college. Neither my mother, nor father had attended college. Most of my siblings hadn't gone past high school. But Maryanne and Jack were my one good link to Joey, so I couldn't allow my insecurities to provoke a pointless argument.

"Doing what?" I'd ask. I'd keep my voice even, use a frank tone. Were there openings for retired drug addicts that I didn't know about?

One time she said, "Don't you think I'd like to go to college too?"

"You should, Maryanne," I said. "I'm enjoying it way more than I thought I would. And your earning potential would increase by getting a degree." My experience deflecting unsolicited criticism in recovery meetings helped keep the conversations civil.

One night shortly before I moved into the dorm, Jack grabbed the phone from Maryanne just as we were ending our conversation. I could hear a muffled discussion as Maryanne held the receiver to her body and then Jack's deep voice was on the line. Other than to say hello, Jack and I rarely spoke to one another.

"Tim," Jack said. "Don't you think it's time you stopped screwing around?"

"Hey, Jack." I said.

I'd known Jack long before Maryanne had moved in with him. We weren't close, but we weren't enemies either. Jack started to explain his difficult financial position, but I didn't catch much of what he said. I could feel a knot tightening somewhere in my chest. For months, the New York City tabloids had been on a campaign to disgrace unforthcoming fathers who had fallen behind in support payments. "Deadbeat Dads," they were called. Some of these men were clearly scofflaws, but the public shaming had made me sensitive to criticism about my small support payments, especially from anyone other than Maryanne.

The phone went silent and I understood Jack was waiting for me to respond.

"I hear you, Jack," I said. "But my hands are tied."

Jack started to balk, but I cut him off.

"I probably shouldn't even tell you this," I said, "but I want to help."

There were two ways to do child support: Either you worked out an amicable agreement, or you went through the courts. Maryanne and I had been using the courts since Joey was two years old. The people at the child support office had warned me never to send money directly to Maryanne. The only way I should send money to them was through the official channels, so that it could be applied to the balance that I owed. "If you want more," I said, "you have to go to the court and request an increase."

The phone went silent again.

I didn't know where that explanation had come from. I'd been feeling shame and growing anger and then suddenly I was explaining child support. In recovery meetings, old timers always told you to pray for the people you were angry at, even if you had been wronged. "You better pray for his ass," they'd say. I understood this to mean that I should try to empathize with the other person. I was amazed at how easily I had slipped into empathy, rather than giving in to anger. Perhaps this was only because Jack hadn't wronged me; on the contrary, he was helping to raise Joey. But, really, he was wrestling with financial problems, just like me. I felt a small glow of pride that I'd said the right thing. As I held the phone to my ear, I jingled the coins in my pocket, and waited to hear what he would say.

Jack sighed.

He apologized for his tone, and I told him to forget it. We traded pleasantries and then said goodnight.

But as soon as we hung up, I felt a rush of anxiety.

I wondered if Maryanne would race to petition the courts for more support, and whether I would ever be able to pay it. If I paid more support, would I still be able to go to school?

I removed the change from my pockets and made short coin stacks on the kitchen table.

I knew if I asked Roger about any of this, he would say that I was powerless over Maryanne, Jack, and anything the support enforcement court might decide. This realization made me feel better. If I was powerless over those things, then there was no sense worrying over them. I would have to depend on myself and my own abilities to manage whatever came up.

I tipped the stacks of coins and they spilled into a messy pile on the table.

* * *

Tess Gallant had pale skin, shoulder-length black hair, and dark red lips.

Dressed entirely in black, she sat at the desk in the front of the room and fixed her coffee, a small paper cup she had pulled from a brown bag. She added sugar and a packet of liquid cream. She slowly stirred. Gazing around the room, she addressed the class.

"This is Fiction 101," she said. I had been attending Hunter College for more than a year and this was my first fiction course.

She told us it was our class and we could do with it what we wanted. Did we want to read? She could assign a book. Did we want to do writing exercises? She knew plenty.

The dozen students in the room sat quietly.

Tess said she thought we'd learn the most about fiction by writing it ourselves and then reading and commenting on one another's work. I loved how self-assured she seemed. She answered questions in an easy, off-hand manner. This wasn't my first creative writing class, but this was the first creative writing class where I saw a writer I wanted to emulate. The other teachers spouted positive aphorisms or focused on grammar. Tess was different. She talked about writing as if it were a way of life. She treated stories as serious business.

I handed in my first story—a pseudo-allegory of heroin addiction that featured a vampire, dumped by his wife—and she glanced at the first page and immediately handed it back. "Genre fiction is fine," she said. "But I can't help you much with it."

I was hurt, disappointed. I asked her what sort of fiction she wanted. Rummaging through her bag, she pulled out an issue of the *New Yorker* magazine.

"Read this," she said. "This is what we do."

*   *   *

Joey was one of the boys standing in the outfield, of that much I was certain, but not much more. All the boys looked alike in their caps and baseball uniforms. I couldn't quite make out which one was my son.

"Is this still the first quarter?" I asked Maryanne.

Maryanne narrowed her eyes at me in disbelief, then grimaced and looked away. Her gaze fixed on the field, she silently shook her head.

I sighed and my gaze wandered.

This was my last visit to Pennsylvania before the new school year began in the fall. I had amassed about half the credits I needed to graduate and decided to focus my efforts in school on writing.

The sun was hot. Dust from the infield wafted into the short bleachers along the third-base line. I left my seat to stand by the batting cage. After each pitch, the umpire barked out a call. Maryanne had invited me to this game for Joey's team. She explained that it was some kind of championship game, how Joey had been recruited by one of the coaches, and that it was an honor for him to be asked to play on the team. I nodded, but didn't really understand what was going on.

In the last year, my visits to Joey had changed in small but fundamental ways. Instead of Joey and me playing catch or going to a movie together, we spent the day at his games—him on the field, me in the stands. Joey played football, basketball, and baseball. He was a talented and graceful athlete, a real natural.

I saw a woman standing on the third base line and recognized her as Grace, one of the cheerleaders from my high-school class. I grinned and walked over near her. We reminisced for a few minutes as the teams changed field positions. She told me she had joined the Navy and been married and divorced since high school. When it came time for me to share my story, I stayed quiet. She took this in stride and we stood next to one another watching the game.

"Why are you here?" Grace asked.

There was a crack and Joey came tearing down the third-base line.

"My son," I said, nodding toward the field. I raised my arms and cheered. "Joey!" I said.

"Jack and Maryanne's boy?" she asked, giving me a confused look.

"Joey is my son," I said.

Her eyes opened wide and she grabbed my forearm with both hands. "Oh, right. Yes!" Grace said. "That's your son. You and Maryanne were together."

I shrugged, smiled.

"I'm so sorry," she said. She took her hand from my forearm, held both her arms in front of her body, and softly chided herself.

"Disgraceful!" A woman barked from a nearby lawn chair. She didn't look our way, but took another sip from her can of beer and spoke loudly enough for her voice to rise above the din on the field and in the stands. "It's just a disgrace!"

I leaned forward to get a better look at this woman. It was another cheerleader from my high school class. "Is that Fanny?" I whispered.

"Yes," Grace said. She grinned and looked embarrassed. "That's Fanny."

"Disgraceful," Fanny said. "Takes off and lets another man raise his child." She took a long draught from her beer and I half expected her to crush the can against her thigh.

Grace whispered, "Don't mind her."

I appreciated her kindness, but I watched the rest of the game alone, from behind the batter's cage, as far away from Fanny as I could get.

Joey went out with his baseball team after the game, and I returned to my mother's house. Relaxing in the living room, I watched television by myself, not paying much attention to the small screen. I felt exhausted and wanted to rest before Joey came to sleep over later.

"Door," my mother said.

Her voice was curt. She stood stiffly and motioned toward the front door with her head.

"What?" I asked. I felt mildly alarmed by her sharp tone.

She looked quickly around the room until she spotted her purse, a large leather bag lying in a pile on an end table. Scooping the purse into her arms, she went into the kitchen without saying another word.

I got up off the couch and went to the front door. Poking my head outside, I found an old friend standing on the front porch.

He grinned at me.

I laughed.

"Sam!" He had long curly dark hair tied into a ponytail and wore a jean jacket with the sleeves pushed back on his sinewy forearms. I hadn't seen him in years, but he hadn't changed a bit.

"Sammy," I said. I stepped onto the porch and let the screen door close behind me. His grin was infectious and I started to chuckle. "You got my mom defending her purse, man."

"I'm sorry," Sam said. His grin faded and he looked contrite. "I'm in recovery!" he said. Sam held up a little key chain and jiggled it like a tiny bell.

"Wow," I said. "Look at you."

"Everyone at the meetings talks about you," Sam said. "You made it in New York City, man. We're all still sweating it out in this dump." He motioned with his hands to indicate all of Steelton.

I felt surprised. Occasionally I went to recovery meetings in this area, but for the most part I reserved my time here for Joey. I asked Sam how it was possible that anyone knew anything about me.

"This is Steelton," Sam laughed. "You can't keep anything secret."

* * *

I loved Tess's classes. At the end of each semester, I'd ask her which nights she planned to teach in the upcoming semester. She would encourage me to attend the classes of a wide range of teachers, to get the most out of my college experience. "Sure, sure," I'd tell her. "But which class do you think *you'll* do next semester?" And then I always made sure to enroll in Tess's class.

My fiction wasn't really fiction at all, but stories loosely based on my life. I wrote about addicts who lost their wives or ended up in crazy drug treatment institutions. Tess took it all in stride. I longed for the little comments she would scribble in the margins of my papers. I always spoke to her after class, usually about my stories. She saved certain comments to share with me at this time, rather than in front of the whole class. If I wrote a clichéd phrase or used a particularly hackneyed image, she would point to it and laugh.

"This right here," she'd say. "This is bullshit."

And I'd take it home and rework it.

She turned me on to her favorite writers (Raymond Carver, Tobias Wolff), who then became my favorite writers. One night after one of her classes, she jotted "THIS BOY'S LIFE" on a scrap of paper and handed it to me.

"Read this book," she said. "Don't watch the movie."

Tobias Wolff's coming-of-age memoir floored me. For days after I read it, I walked around campus with it in my hand, hoping to find someone with whom to discuss it with. His characters were the people I grew up with and wanted so badly to escape from: the petty stepfathers, the overbearing disciplinarians and resourceful mothers, and so many clever children trapped in a small dying town. Yet his story—the way he told it—so utterly engrossed me. I finished it quickly—no more than a day or two of whipping it out whenever I had a few moments, and then one long draught on a sleepless night. Somehow the combination of familiar characters and engrossing story filled me with hope. If Wolff could make such an engaging story from the likes of his life, then anything seemed possible. Who could say? The universe could suddenly open up and anything at all might happen.

*   *   *

Maryanne wanted me to sit at her dining room table. She had sent Joey upstairs to brush his teeth and pack an overnight bag; he would be sleeping over with me at my mother's house. At this point I had about three-quarters of the credits I needed to graduate from Hunter.

Jack was already at the table. He nodded and smiled. Maryanne pulled a long white envelope from her purse and passed it to me. The top had been ripped open and there was a cellophane window on the front. "What's this?" I asked.

"Read it," she said.

I looked at Jack, then Maryanne.

I could hear Joey dashing from room to room upstairs and then the sound of the bathroom faucet running. The letter was addressed to Maryanne. I didn't recognize the return address or the name of the company. Inside the envelope, I found a single pink legal-size form filled with figures and smallish print. No sooner had I glanced at it, than Maryanne started to talk. She began telling me about the cost of Joey's health care, which surprised me. He seemed so healthy. There were so many large amounts listed on the form, it was hard to determine how much was on the line. I mentioned to Maryanne that I hadn't even considered the cost of Joey's health care. I had always assumed that her coverage from work covered Joey.

"For the most part it does," Maryanne said. "But we need more help."

"Have you petitioned the courts for an increase?" I asked. I raised my head from the form, half-afraid to hear her answer.

"New York City support authority sucks," Maryanne said. "The out-of-state claims department is a nightmare."

"We can't get through," Jack said. "We've been at it forever."

I felt relieved. And then I felt guilty for feeling relieved.

I turned back to the form in my hand and then I saw it. In the very bottom margin of the page in the tiniest print: THIS IS NOT A BILL.

*　*　*

I spotted Tess striding across the street.

We had a class together in a few hours. Picking up my pace, I fell into step next to her and she grinned. Once after class, I had told her about my drug history and then she told me about her own. She had done heroin recreationally for a few years. I didn't even know you could do heroin that way. We bonded over our past history of substance abuse.

Tess pointed us toward a small grocery near the school.

She was telling me something about the pitfalls of working as an adjunct. I followed her into the store and then shadowed her in the aisles. As we waited in the checkout line, she told me about a plan to kick-start her publishing career that involved living in an art colony in the woods somewhere in Southern California.

I stood with her, half-listening, lost in my own thoughts.

"How was your trip to Pennsylvania?" she asked.

I didn't mind sharing with Tess how inadequate I felt as a parent. I could tell she didn't seem particularly interested in discussing parenting, which made me feel confident about discussing it with her. She wouldn't weigh in with heavy-handed judgments or bleak pronouncements. Mostly she just listened, which was alright by me.

"Joey did his first communion," I said. "I got him a bike."

In New York City, my problems with old high-school classmates or drug-addict friends in Steelton seemed remote, an intellectual exercise. The real issue was how to show up for Joey from so far away. People often gave me suggestions, some of which worked better than others. Send mail, someone said. Kids love to get personal mail. Or, come up with talking points for phone calls, someone else suggested. This idea was a real winner for getting something from those long-distance phone calls, which could be exceptionally painful given the monosyllabic replies of an elementary-school boy.

"You know what you should be thinking about," Tess said. She had stopped and turned to look at me. People drifted around us on the sidewalk. "Take your cue from fiction for kids. There is almost always this one character in every book—the Crazy Aunt."

"*Crazy Aunt*?" I said. We started to make our way up Lexington.

"The Crazy Aunt is an outsider—she is someone who sweeps in with an absolutely different worldview and offers the protagonist a different set of options. These are options that no one else in her world could possibly offer her, because they've never gone outside their own little world."

"Crazy Aunt," I said. My voice was flat, skeptical.

"It's not always an aunt," Tess said. "That's just what they call the archetype. Almost every book I read as a girl had a Crazy Aunt character."

"So the Crazy Aunt could be, like, a Crazy Uncle?" I asked.

Tess had grown animated and excited with her analogy, but I wasn't sure how to relate to a female character, especially one who sounded like she had bats in her belfry.

"Dude," Tess said, "the Crazy Aunt is the hero."

Her voice sounded a little defensive.

I grinned. "I guess I was hoping for an archetype a little more *badass*."

Tess shook her head and chuckled.

She never gave me any other advice about how to relate to my son, and she left for the West Coast shortly after that semester. Less than ten years later, I would discover that she'd written an amazing novel, an instant bestseller that would receive much critical acclaim and be turned into a major motion picture.

Her perseverance had finally paid off—and it paid off big.

I had teased Tess that afternoon on Lexington Avenue, but what she suggested about using literary devices to resolve family situations had wormed its way into my mind. More than learning how to write, I was learning how to use literature to sustain myself, to help me to imagine a new world for myself, even as I muddled through my own mundane realities. Tess had helped to open my mind and engage my imagination. When I needed to be at my most creative as a parent and father, I clung to her suggestion, offered up on a busy New York City sidewalk on a bright spring day.

And that suggestion—coupled with my own willingness to use it—would pay off.

And pay off big.

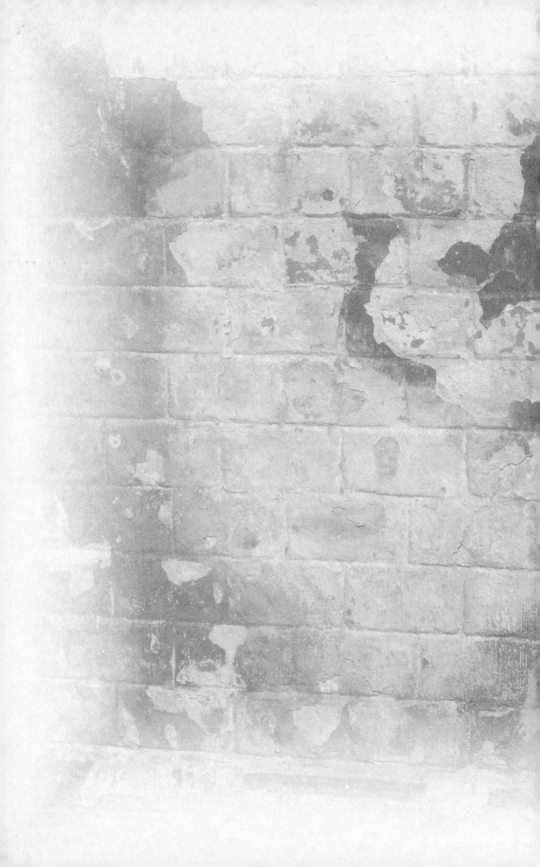

CHAPTER 7

HUMILITY

Joey was waiting for my call.

I sat in my dorm room, listening to the hiss and screech of the modem as it searched for a connection to the Internet. I had been putting off the call to Joey most of the spring and into the summer. When I wasn't in school or at work, I was usually in front of my computer in my dorm room, connecting to an Internet community hosted somewhere on a server in Washington State. By throwing myself into a virtual world, I could escape my own reality here in New York. Only a few credits shy of the number I needed to graduate, I would finish school in the spring and then have to move out of the dorm. I cringed at the thought of standing around in mortarboard and gown with an auditorium full of twenty-something students and their smiling, proud parents, and I didn't even want to think about what I was going to do after school.

The modem settled down, and I logged in. I scanned the list of who else was logged on. I was looking for Holly, a woman from Seattle whom I had been pursuing hard all summer. She had flown into DC on a business trip and then came up here to spend the Fourth of July holiday with me. We held hands on the deck of the Staten Island ferry and watched fireworks explode over the Statue of Liberty.

Everything was changing.

My employment landscape had completely transformed—Dean Bernstein had moved on, Mrs. Shannon had died. I'd found a job providing security at a small, posh shop on Park Avenue, near school. I had to wear a tie and stand discreetly among the racks for most of the day. I didn't like it. Once as I stood in the corner, an elderly woman approached and turned her back to me, the zipper on her dress open to her waist. "Dear?" she said.

Holly was not logged in. I knew our relationship had real potential when she mentioned that her mother had long been after her to attend recovery meetings, but for a different program than the one I was in. I was excited that this was something we could share. I broke the Internet connection and considered calling her at home instead. Calculating the time difference, I tried to determine what she might be doing that very minute.

I considered finally making the call to Joey and my gut clenched up.

He didn't even realize the call was coming, but he had been waiting for it all summer long, if not his entire life. He deserved a visit, but I knew that was out of the question. I had no idea how to tell him what I had to say and looking into his little blue eyes as I said it seemed too great a challenge.

I picked up the phone and dialed Joey's number.

I hoped his mother would answer. Tell me he wasn't available, so I could task her with giving him the news. Instead he picked up on the second ring, and we finally spoke.

"What's up?" Joey asked. "Where you been?"

I chuckled nervously and made small talk. Now that Joey was ten, I had become expert at keeping our conversations moving forward on the phone. I said the things we usually said and then after a few minutes, I said, "Son. We should talk."

I told him school was coming to a close for me.

I knew he would ask the same question he always asked, Where would I live? By this I know he meant where *in Steelton* would I live. Would I get an apartment on Front Street or rent one of the row homes on Cottage Hill? I had known for a long time that I could never live in Steelton again, but I hadn't told him. First, I didn't know what would happen. I could relapse. I had never had recovery last this long and didn't want to have a difficult conversation about something that might end up being a moot point. Second, I kept hoping something would happen, a better solution would present itself.

"Where are you going to live?" he asked, just like he always did. But this time, his voice was cautious, uncertain. I hated myself for causing that tremor in his voice.

"Seattle," I said. "I'm going to move to Washington State."

The phone went quiet and I gave him time to consider this new information. The plan was to move to Seattle over the Christmas break and forward my remaining course work to the school by mail. I only had a few writing classes left and all of my professors had agreed to the plan.

"Seattle?" he asked. "Where is Seattle?"

I hadn't expected this question.

"The Pacific Northwest," I said. "Near Alaska."

"Alaska!" His voice sounded outraged and frightened. I could have kicked myself for using such a remote-sounding place to make my point.

I tried to keep my tone even. I didn't completely understand why I knew I shouldn't live in Steelton, but I recognized the feeling of dread I felt every time I considered that option. I explained about Holly, how much I cared for her. I didn't try to explain about any crazy fears or nonsense about standing around in mortarboards. I promised I would bring Holly to come meet him in Steelton before I left for Seattle.

Joey cut me off, his voice sounding indignant and sad. "I thought you would live in Steelton," he said. "I thought you'd get a pickup truck and I'd sit up front. I thought we'd ride around together. Go to movies and the Harrisburg East Mall." His voice cracked as he said this last part about movies and the mall and then he was silent.

The phone went quiet.

I pinched the bridge of my nose and held the phone against the side of my head; it was all I could do to keep from placing the phone in its cradle and racing out of the room. I blew air noisily out of my mouth and felt hollow inside.

I told him I just couldn't do it. I tried to think of something else to say, but I had nothing. I said that I had to go. And then I hung up.

* * *

Ginny Romano listened to me prattle nervously. She was one of the professors who had agreed to take my remaining coursework from Seattle by mail. We were reviewing logistics, and she had asked me a simple question: "Why Seattle?"

Her question caught me off guard and I grinned like an oaf.

"I met a woman who lives in Seattle," I said.

I felt foolish. Earlier that week, one of my classmates had asked me about the job market in Seattle and with much chagrin I realized I knew absolutely nothing. People who weren't recovering addicts probably made big life decisions in a completely different manner. Or maybe I was just an idiot. To save face, I blurted out some of the logistical challenges associated with the move and how I planned to deal with them.

Ginny was a small woman with dark hair and pleasant face. She liked to tell stories about growing up in an Italian neighborhood on the tough streets of Hoboken. During lectures, she might shove her blouse sleeves up her forearms and shake her fist to look menacing. If my mom had a Ph.D., she would be just like Ginny—tough and proud of her ethnicity.

"My son is terribly disappointed," I said. "He wants me to live with him in Steelton." I hadn't intended to say anything about Joey, but I had been talking about challenges and it just came out of my mouth.

Ginny's expression changed.

She sat forward and her brow furrowed. "You can't do this," she said. "He's your child. You're his father. You can't just move to the other side of the country."

As soon as she said it, I knew it was true. This was the very thought that had been nagging at me all summer, unspoken. Ginny had given the idea a voice and true weight. My shoulders slumped forward and I hung my head.

"I know," I said.

I had been trying to present a cheerful, optimistic exterior. I wanted to inspire confidence, but now all that pretense was gone. I kept my head down as Ginny spoke and didn't catch much of what else she was saying. All I heard was a dull indictment booming in my mind, like the beat of a distant bass drum.

I shook my head and whispered a response, repeated it over and over, and each time I said it, it came out a bit louder, until I was finally speaking it in a normal tone of voice. "I can't go back," I said. "I can't go back."

I hazarded a quick look up at Ginny. My eyes were wet and I was grinning. I felt ridiculous and wished I could articulate the utter certainty I felt that moving to Steelton would be the death of me. Instead I said, "I should go."

Ginny stood with me. "Wait," she said. "Wait."

I turned back.

"It's okay," she said. "It's okay."

She looked unsure of herself for a beat and then she spread her arms wide. "Hug," she said. It wasn't a command, but it wasn't a question either.

I sniffed. Some recovery programs are all about the hug. In others, nothing but a firm handshake will do. I have always been more in the handshake camp, but I crossed the room and put my arms around Ginny. Her head came up to about my chest. I felt her hands pat my back and I gave a big exhalation that felt wonderful.

The next day in Ginny's class I sat toward the back of the room. Our encounter during her office hours had left me feeling vulnerable and exposed. I half expected her to back out of our agreement for the following semester. Why should she want to help me now that she knew I was moving 3,000 miles from Joey?

The class was looking at portraits of dysfunctional families in literature or something. It was a good selection for a fall semester that didn't offer much. Ginny was leading an impromptu discussion about a book that wasn't on the syllabus, but involved a mother who had been abused as a child and then felt that she had to leave her own child in foster care. Ginny leaned casually on the edge of the desk as she discussed this text. In the context of the class, the discussion made perfect sense. A few students recoiled from the character's predicament.

Ginny stood so she could see all the way into the back of the room, where I sat. I felt raw, exposed, with nowhere to hide. I cast my eyes down and stared at my twitching hands.

"Some things," she said slowly, "can at first appear selfish, but might actually be the most reasonable course of action." When she said those words, I looked back at her to see what the expression was on her face. Ginny was gazing right at me, waiting for me to look up.

"No one," she said, "can judge another's motivations."

I could feel emotion welling up at the back of my throat. I dropped my head and waited for it to pass. I thought about our talk in her office, all the feelings that had come up. And as I recalled the feeling of her comforting hug, another idea took shape in my mind—Ginny Romano was almost exactly the same height and size as my mother.

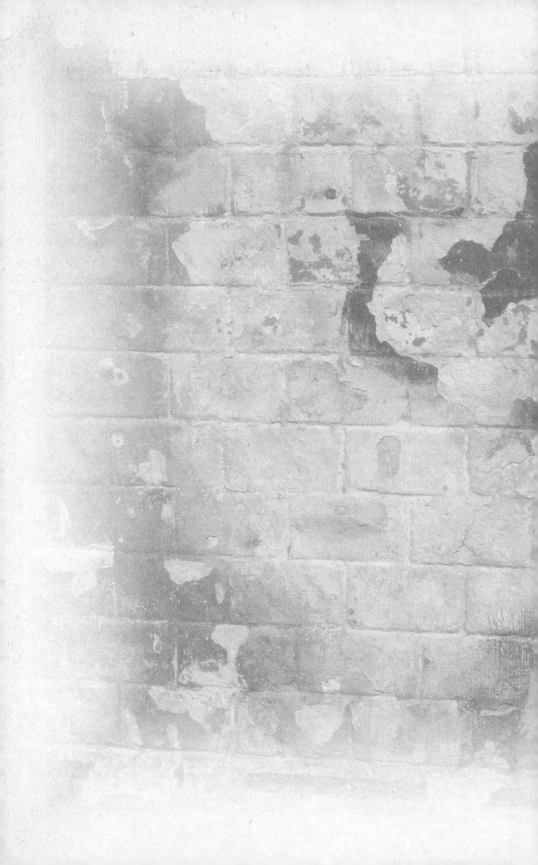

CHAPTER 8

BROTHERLY LOVE

Maryanne hosted a small party for Joey and his friends at her house.

Holly and I had been invited at the last minute, an act of kindness for out-of-town guests. When I left New York, I'd checked out of the dorm and shipped most of my belongings to the address where Holly had been staying in Seattle. My things were already there, and Holly, as I'd promised Joey, had come east to meet him before flying back to Seattle with me. This visit was my big goodbye. Holly begged off the party, but I sat at the dining room table, pushing my ice cream around with a spoon. So far Holly and I had been to a movie with Joey and we had plans to take him to Baltimore to see the Orioles play. Joey had seemed shy with Holly, but she was doing her best to draw him out.

Maryanne stood in the kitchen doorway and announced a movie for the boys to watch. We'd just finished our cake and a raucous cheer went up. Boys drew themselves up from around the dining room table and from their perches on chairs and sofas in the living room. The kids moved downstairs to watch the movie with Jack, a loud herd of boys stomping and hooting down the stairwell. Maryanne carried dirty plates from the dining room to the kitchen. I wanted to make amends to her before I left for Seattle and this was my big shot.

In recovery programs, making amends is huge. Everyone who has any amount of recovery time has an amends story. I had only ever made amends with my mother. We'd been at her house, sitting at the kitchen table. She had filled my cup with freshly brewed coffee and I started off hesitantly, faltering over my words. As the coffee pot hovered over my mug, Mom listened with her head cocked. When she grasped what I was telling her, she dismissed it with a wave of the pot and then darted across the room. I was surprised. In the meetings, the stories about amends always seemed to work out a little more eloquently, a little more heartfelt.

I must have looked hurt. Mom returned the pot to the machine and raced back to me. She put her hand over mine.

"You're fine," she said. "That's all in the past. Let's just forget it."

"There's a financial part," I told Mom, who had grown up poor in the Great Depression and knew the value of a buck. "I can pay you back for the money I stole."

"You got money?" Mom asked. She let go my hand and straightened her back.

"Well, no," I said. "Not yet." I looked down into the blackness of my coffee mug.

"A regular Rockefeller," Mom said wryly.

I looked up and she was grinning.

"I'd pay you," I said. My voice sounded more wounded than I felt.

"You just keep doing what you're doing," Mom said. She stroked my hand again. "That's all I want from you."

But here at Maryanne's party for Joey, making amends didn't seem so straightforward.

I collected a short stack of dirty dishes and carried them into the kitchen where Maryanne stood, loading the dishwasher.

"Aren't you going to watch the movie with the boys?" Maryanne asked. The kitchen felt unnaturally quiet without the boys' raucous noise. She moved to the refrigerator, opened the door, and stood rearranging bottles and jars inside.

"Already seen it," I said. "Let me help you clean up."

I set the dishes down near the sink, and stood with my hands at my sides feeling clumsy. I didn't really know where to start. Financial restitution was a big part of making the amends, but money was such a divisive issue for Maryanne and me. I tried to calculate how much I might owe her, but it was hard to find a total. How many times had I dipped into her purse for money? Did the lies I told about where my paycheck had gone count toward restitution?

I looked at Maryanne and grinned.

She darted across the kitchen. I put a dirty plate into the dishwasher and followed her across the room.

"Maryanne, before I go, there's something I wanted to say to you."

I waited for her to look at me, but she kept her head turned toward the cupboards. I gathered my thoughts for the next big push into the unknown. She stole a glance past the cupboard door toward me. I was drumming my fingertips nervously on my lips.

She slammed the cupboard door and bolted into the dining room.

"Maryanne, wait," I said. I moved to follow her, feeling a little annoyed.

We were almost out of the kitchen when Maryanne spun around, and I had to pull up short to keep from crashing into her.

"Tim," she said. "Enough."

She pointed her finger at my throat like a weapon. "I have to tell you," she said. "I am very happy with Jack. Very happy." She made a little karate-chop gesture with her hand. "We have a life together," she said. She stopped, held her arms out, and glanced around the room.

"A life together," she said.

I cocked my head uncertainly.

"Do you know what I'm telling you?" Maryanne asked.

I shook my head in confusion, even though everything she was saying seemed obvious.

"Jack and I are together," Maryanne said. She made a gesture with her hands like an umpire declaring a base runner safe.

"Together," she repeated. Her voice snapped like a flag in the wind.

Nodding her head, she turned and continued clearing the dining room table.

I stood in the kitchen doorway with nothing to say. I'd never heard about amends stories that went this poorly. I decided I had better postpone my work with Maryanne for some other time.

* * *

I came down the stairs at my mother's house.

I had been down these stairs millions of times. I knew which of the wooden steps would squeak and the cool firmness of the milled rail. My visit was almost over and I was pleased with how well-received Holly had been. My brothers and sisters seemed to be making a special effort to drop in at my mom's house to see us off.

As I reached the bottom of the stairs, I saw a family portrait hanging on the wall opposite the landing, and pulled up short. This family portrait was from the 60s, with all seven siblings and my parents. We had many portraits like these, but this one was special. Most of our portraiture was from department stores, but this one had been done in a professional studio, probably an extravagance by young parents celebrating the completion of a large family. The lighting was warm, clearly defining each child's head. All of our eyes were looking up and forward to some unknown point on the horizon.

When I was a boy, I'd cut my face from this portrait.

I stopped and stared into the eyes of my childhood face for a few minutes. I could hear my mother, Holly, and the others in the kitchen. I wondered if I was mistaken about this portrait, but the soft pastel colorizing made this photograph unmistakable. Someone had given it a new wooden frame, glass, and matting from the craft store.

When I was ten or twelve, I had always felt different, strange, excluded. Snooping around, I'd found this portrait on the back porch where I knew I wasn't allowed. When the idea to cut my face from the picture popped into my head, it felt right. Exactly right. I knew this was one of my mother's favorite portraits. I knew she had stored it in the chest on the porch behind the bathroom to keep it safe. But I also knew I had to cut it. How could I not? I used a small pair of steel scissors with black handles. I remember wielding the scissors so carefully, not wanting to ruin the rest of the picture, but then—halfway through the act—realizing that trying to protect the others was foolish: You can't remove a boy from the picture without ruining the whole.

Holly laughed. I followed the noise into the kitchen.

"Mom, where did you get that picture in the living room?" I asked.

Mom was holding her ever-present coffee pot, explaining something to Holly as she turned to me. "Which one?" she asked.

"The family portrait at the bottom of the stairs?" I said. "I thought all of those portraits were. . . ." My voice trailed off and I wasn't sure how to phrase the question. She had been so disappointed with me when she found the damaged portrait.

"Ruined?" I finally said.

Mom sighed. "They were ruined," she said.

Turning to Holly, Mom said, "This one was a challenge to raise."

"This picture looks okay to me," I said.

"Look again," Mom said.

I returned to the landing and Mom followed.

"Looks good," I said.

Mom flipped on the overhead light. I leaned in closer to examine.

"Look at your head," Mom said.

I had to look at it from the side, but finally I saw the faint cut lines around where my head was in the picture. There was another picture of me pasted behind the picture of the rest of the family.

"What did you do here?" I asked. "How did you do this?"

"That's one of your elementary school pictures," Mom said.

I could see the head on my shoulders was a little older, out of place. But it wasn't too noticeable. The head and eyes were pointing in the right direction. The backgrounds from both pictures seemed to match.

Holly had followed us into the room. Mom turned to her and explained the challenge of getting me back into the picture.

"How did you get the backgrounds to match up?" I asked.

"A little shoe polish," Mom said.

I laughed.

"Cheap?" Mom asked. She was asking me to evaluate her work.

Now that I knew the story and the light was on, I could see the portrait was a little Frankenstein. "Not cheap," I said. "No."

I felt connected to my family in a way I hadn't in many years.

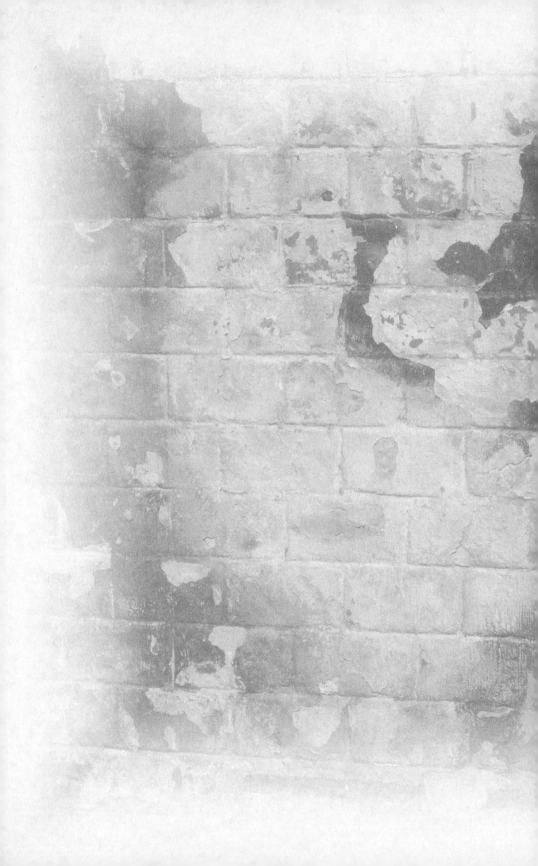

CHAPTER 9

JUSTICE

I found a small room above a Thai restaurant on Pike Street in Seattle. The bathroom was at the end of the hallway, shared by half a dozen or so other residents. Most days were wet, gray, and cold. Some days I woke up in a panic and thought, "What have I done?" I couldn't afford to let myself slip into the dregs of depression, so I sought out a new recovery sponsor and a therapist willing to see me on a sliding-scale rate. I finished all of my remaining course work and got a job on a landscaping crew. Winter was mild. One crisp day in February, I walked out of my room and into the morning sunshine. Looking south, I spied my first ever glimpse of Mount Rainier, a huge snow-covered mountain squatting on the horizon. I hadn't even realized it was there.

I applied for a writing job, documenting software products at a company located in Seattle's Eastside. The newspaper advertisement said I needed writing samples, so I brought a few poems, one of which contained the word, "goddamn." One of the interviewers, a bald man about my age wearing cowboy boots, said that although he didn't mind the word, he didn't think it appropriate for any future interviews. I hadn't even considered it. The hiring manager asked me what salary I expected, which was one more thing I hadn't thought out. I told her the first number that came into my mind: "Twenty," I said. She smiled and said she would give me twenty-four. I knew I had negotiated poorly, but I still had to resist the impulse to laugh and whisper incredulously, "*Thousand*?"

Holly and I moved into an apartment on Boren Avenue and began talking about marriage. We both went to recovery meetings in our respective programs. My sliding-scale therapist, an older woman with a carefully arranged coiffure of gray curls, felt that my move to Seattle and my love for Holly were all misguided responses to fear and anxiety. She wrung her hands and spoke gravely. "You must not marry this woman," she said.

I ditched the therapist and planned a lovely service in our apartment.

A pastor friend Holly knew from her recovery program agreed to officiate. Holly's younger brother flew up from California. One of my new recovery friends was best man. Holly looked radiant in a long, floral dress.

I stood in the kitchen with a few friends waiting for the service to start. Pastor John called from the living room for us to get going. A great wave of nervous energy passed over me and my mouth dried up. I swallowed hard and watched our friends mill toward the other end of the apartment where the ceremony would take place. I glanced at Holly who looked fresh and delicious. I started to inch away from her toward the bathroom, but she took my elbow in her hand.

"I'll be right in," I said. "I just need some water."

I tried to pull away, but she pressed her warm body against mine. Looking into her eyes, I could see she felt anxious too. She was about my height, and she leaned her head toward my ear.

I hoped she would kiss me right then, tell me everything would be alright. Instead she whispered, "You're not going anywhere, bastard. Get in the living room."

* * *

The engineers I met in software development were often shy and socially awkward people. I was exceptionally good at interviewing them—perhaps my recovery experience working with shy and awkward newcomers helped. In my first year, I discovered the lowest-paid writer in the group was me. I asked for and received almost a fifty percent raise.

Holly and I settled into a routine, but marriage was a difficult transition for me. One night I came home from work, grabbed some of the dinner Holly had made, and sat down to eat. We lived in a large studio apartment with a small separate kitchenette and bathroom; the TV, my desk and computer, and our bed all fit in one room lined with large leaded glass windows overlooking Boren Street. This was the room where we typically ate our meals. I turned on the TV, sat at my desk and fired up the computer. After the modem screamed to life, I kicked off a few USENET porn downloads, then moved to sit at the end of the bed, watch TV, and eat.

Holly came out of the kitchen with her own plate of food. She stood poking her fork into her pasta and watching the program on TV.

"This is really good," I said, pointing to my plate.

"What are you doing," Holly asked.

"Watching TV," I said. I was confused. What did she think I was doing?

"No, on the computer," she said. "What are you doing over there?" She pointed with her fork.

"That," I said. "I'm downloading porn."

"You can't be downloading porn," she said. "You're married."

"Are you kidding?" I asked.

She was not kidding.

I had many things to learn about living with a woman in a committed relationship. It wasn't easy, even if we were both in recovery.

During this time, I sought out Dave, my new sponsor in Seattle, who fit most of my requirements for a sponsor: male, many years of recovery, with something vaguely fatherly in his manner. He was also gay and didn't know much about married women.

"She won't let me download porn," I complained.

"Wow," Dave said. He wore his silver hair clipped short, which gave him a distinguished look and offered a certain weight to any suggestion he made, no matter how obvious. "Maybe take it a day at a time?"

Thankfully, I had no clue about all the things that I didn't know.

Two years after we married, Holly discovered she was having twins. I was overjoyed.

As Holly's belly grew, I learned from Joey that Maryanne was also pregnant again. Maryanne and Jack had had a child together just as I was moving to Seattle, and now they were having another. Both our families would increase by two in the short amount of time since I had moved.

Holly and I moved to an apartment on the Eastside. The suburbs seemed like a good place to raise a family and I would be closer to work. One day I returned from work and found an official-looking letter from the Seattle Department of Child Support in the evening mail.

Maryanne had petitioned the court for more support.

I'd known this day would come. I earned a lot more now than I had when the current amount had been set. But I also had more responsibility than ever before. I remembered how frightened and powerless I'd felt standing before the judge in the Bronx. I thought of the screaming man in the court room, his eyes wide, his face livid.

I didn't know what to do. Holly declined to weigh in. Dave turned the question back to me and asked what I thought I ought to do.

I hired a lawyer.

*   *   *

The lawyer called me at work.

I had declined to attend the support hearing and asked her to represent me instead. She was calling to report back on what had happened during the hearing, which was held in Pennsylvania and which she had attended by phone. She told me that my child support payment would increase, but it would increase by less than the amount originally proposed. Her voice was buoyant.

For some reason, I didn't feel happy. Halfway through our conversation I realized how discordant our voices were and apologized. What did I have to be upset about? I couldn't imagine. I agreed that she'd gotten me the best outcome we could have hoped for, and I thanked her for her help. After we hung up, I couldn't shake the unsettled feeling. When the twins were born, Holly's mother traveled up from California and stayed at our apartment. We had much to figure out, the least of which was how to breastfeed two hungry babies. The children were a few weeks early but healthy enough to leave the hospital. Holly sat on the couch with a U-shaped pillow in her lap. Her mom and I hovered over her as she jockeyed the children's large bald heads near her equally large, swollen breasts. Peering down from above us, you would have been reminded of a football huddle. We were the hungriest, most sleep-deprived, and confused football team in all the land. After two weeks, Holly's mom said she was heading back to California, and I had to hide my shock and dismay. Who would raise these children?

The first few months were difficult, but eventually Holly and I fell into a groove.

One afternoon I called Joey for a routine check-in and Maryanne answered. I asked her about her new baby and she asked after my twins. I asked her if the new support checks had started making their way through the system, though I was pretty sure they had. She said they had. And then I asked her about the support hearing. Had she even attended?

"Of course I went," Maryanne said. Her tone went sharp.

I swallowed and felt the muscles in my shoulders and back go tense.

"I don't have money for a lawyer," Maryanne said. "But I had to face the one you hired."

I looked around the room, searching for some place to hide. If you've ever known someone as long as I have known Maryanne, you learn their body language and mannerisms well enough that you can tell how they'll react just by hearing the tone of their voice. I could tell that Maryanne had her hand on her hip, her body pitched just a little forward, to give a weight to her words that her slim frame couldn't otherwise manage. Her face was a little flushed, her blue eyes sparkling-hot. If she wasn't holding the phone in her hand, she'd be wagging her finger in my face.

I held the phone to my ear and listened. I said nothing.

Maryanne was fierce, especially if she was fighting for something just. But I could hear anxiety and fear in her voice as she recounted the hearing. I had put her in the exact position I was trying to avoid: fighting a nameless, faceless bureaucracy, where it wasn't so much whether you were right or wrong that mattered, as how well you could present yourself.

She finally slowed down.

I felt awful. I didn't know if I should tell Maryanne how bad I felt or if I should just apologize. Finally, I just said that I didn't realize she would have to defend herself against my lawyer.

"That must have been hard," I said.

Maryanne sighed. "Damn right."

* * *

Holly said we should look for a house.

Each night after work we loaded the children into the car and drove around the Eastside. We found a small ranch house in a neighborhood that had been built for Boeing employees but was now a mix of working class, retirees, and young professionals. A greenbelt behind the house held a stand of old fir trees that would sway in the high winds.

At the bank, Holly and I sat behind the desk of a financial officer who gazed into her computer monitor and told us what documents we would need. "I'm seeing some liens against Tim here," she said. When she looked across the desk at me, she lowered her head and peered at me over her glasses.

"*Liens*?" I said. I wasn't sure what the word meant.

"Liens in Pennsylvania, New York, and Washington," she said.

"Child support," I said. I had never caught up from the time in New York when I had let it accrue.

"How much is it?" I asked.

The bank officer said a number in the tens of thousands. I was astonished. I looked at Holly who was already looking at me.

"That's too much," I said. "No way do I owe that much."

"You could be right," the bank officer said. She explained that liens were judgments against me and that they would all have to be dealt with for the financing on the house to go through.

"How do I deal with the liens?" I asked.

"Most people pay them," she said.

But I didn't have tens of thousands of dollars. Even though we were both working, Holly and I didn't even have enough for a down payment for a house. We were trying to get a house financed by the veterans' administration with no money down.

"Call them," the bank officer said. "See what you can find out."

I called the Child Support office in Washington and learned that I would have to pay off any arrearage to lift the judgment. I asked about the liens in the other states. Washington had no idea, but assured me that they were the final authority for the order with my son. I called Pennsylvania and waited on hold for hours. When I finally got through, Pennsylvania told me to call Washington for any questions or problems. New York didn't even bother to answer. The phone just rang and rang and rang and nobody ever picked up.

Each state has a certain type of number for its cases. If you don't have a state code for your case, you're an aberration to the system, and you are put on hold. When I would reach someone, they would have no idea what to make of my story. Working with them to understand the problem was often tedious work. "Well, let me ask you this," one clerk said. "Do you have any *other children* in Pennsylvania or New York?" She stressed the words "other children" as if she were reciting some magic incantation that would somehow unlock the puzzle.

"No ma'am," I said. "Just the one boy."

The best I could determine was that a judgment was opened in each state during the time I lived in the state. Although authority for support would follow me to the new state, the previous state would keep its judgments open. Fortunately I had habitually hoarded all of the paperwork that had ever been sent to me by a support office. I scoured through every scrap of official letterhead for phone numbers different from the main public phone number each state publicized for parents who needed help with child support. I would get up early in the morning to call back east just as the offices were opening for the day. At night before I went to sleep I would fantasize about hiring a lawyer to cut through the red tape, but I knew I couldn't afford to pay anyone for this many billable hours. I felt like I was paying some karmic price for the way I handled my support hearing. I was powerless against this huge bureaucracy, but my own feelings of inadequacy and shame were the real behemoths that I struggled against. I resolved to handle my situation with good cheer. All I could do was this: Get up early and make phone calls. Speak sincerely and without scorn to the people who answered. Pray.

Finally I made headway.

I learned that the lien in Pennsylvania would go away automatically when the arrears in Washington were paid. Only New York stood in my way. No one in Pennsylvania or Washington understood why New York still had a lien. One morning I called the New York office in my pajamas, rubbing the sleep from my eyes. After only a few rings, I got an answer and had my call redirected to a woman with a soft tremor in her voice. I explained my situation and she did something no other state employee had ever done before—she gave me her name and her phone extension. She told me she would look into it.

And she did.

In a few weeks, I went to closing with my wife and about eight thousand dollars. We paid the arrearage and got the house. For the first time in my life, I was up-to-date on child support and living in my own home.

CHAPTER 10

PERSEVERANCE

Over the next five years, my relationship with Joey consisted of many phone calls. I tried to visit Pennsylvania every year. On one trip, Joey helped me carry our big double-wide stroller up some concrete stairs and into the Zoo, so we could visit with his family. Most of my brothers and sisters had married and started families of their own, and so my extended family in Pennsylvania included teachers, police officers, a preacher, and even a used-car dealer. Everyone pitched in to help Joey, and I felt grateful. Every once in a while Maryanne or my mom would call on me to mediate some dispute that involved my son, but for the most part I felt useless, watching as others met my son's emotional needs.

During his senior year in high school, Joey grew. And grew. I heard about this change from Maryanne and my family, but it was hard for me to grasp.

He had always been an athletic child. Jack had always joked about how much Joey ate. Maryanne liked to joke about how quickly he outgrew his shoes. I heard this new chatter about his dimensions and relegated it to the kind of things people say to carry a conversation along.

"He's getting really big," Maryanne might say.

Or Mom might say, "What are they feeding that boy?"

One afternoon Joey and I were talking on the phone and with great pride he told me he had shattered another boy's facemask at football practice.

I wasn't sure how to respond.

"Wow," I said. "Do you think it was a defective facemask?"

"Dad," Joey said. "It wasn't defective, it was a facemask. You know—a facemask? Like, to protect your face." I could hear deep disappointment in his voice.

"Well, how did you break it, son?"

Joey sighed. "I have to hang up now," he said.

I could hear his aversion for our conversation, but felt helpless to change it. I called back a few days later and Maryanne answered. Instead of immediately calling Joey, she settled into a conversation with me. "What you don't realize," Maryanne said, "is that he's big as a house. He's even bigger than Jack."

"Bigger than Jack?" I said. "He's over six feet?"

I couldn't believe it. Jack was taller than me.

Maryanne laughed.

"They love him on the football team," she said. "He just runs right over all the other boys."

When Joey got on the phone, all was forgiven. I told him that I had no idea he had gotten so big. He said his mom had already explained all that to him. We laughed together, and I was happy we figured it out, but I also felt discouraged. In some ways my relationship with Joey remained small and claustrophobic. With my four-year-old twins, I had found a comfortable parenting rhythm. With my seventeen-year-old big-as-a-man child, I was still struggling to find my groove.

*   *   *

I took Holly and the twins to Pennsylvania for Joey's high school graduation. He drove out to meet us at my brother's house in an old Japanese compact car. I went outside to greet him. He didn't so much slip out of the car as peel himself out of it. It was like watching circus clowns emerging from a tiny car. He just kept coming and coming. He seemed to have somehow folded himself into the driver's seat. One of his hands was on the door, the other on the roof, and the entire vehicle listed to the driver side as he got out. I was amazed. Even a little frightened. Who was this large person?

I stood and stared at him.

He grinned, and then I could see my little boy.

"Damn, son," I said. "I'm going to have to start calling you Joe. You're no Joey anymore"

"Hey Pop," Joey said.

We did our first awkward man-hug.

We went over the plans for the weekend. Maryanne was having a pig roast for him and his friends at her new house in Chambers Hill, a few miles outside of Steelton in the suburbs of Hershey. We were all invited.

At the pig roast, Holly and I stood in Maryanne and Jack's suburban backyard on a crisp, spring day. Joey sat at a picnic table with his teenage friends. He introduced me and Holly, but I didn't want to inhibit their fun, so I spent most of my time with the adult guests. I chatted with Maryanne's mother and stepfather, whom I hadn't seen in ages. Jack had invited some of his employees and their families, one of whom was a woman I had been in treatment with back in the '80s. She stood sipping beer from a plastic cup. As we reminisced, I couldn't help but notice how hard the years had been on her.

Another guest was a wizened man in tattered sneakers who grew animated as I approached him. We chatted for a few minutes. He acted like he knew me, but I struggled to place his face. He had light blue eyes buried in a bed of crags and wrinkles.

"You know who I am?" he asked.

"You do look familiar," I said. I smiled and shrugged.

"Matt," he said. "Maryanne's little brother."

I was astonished.

Matt had somehow managed to transform himself from a gawky teenager into a little old man. He was at least ten years younger than I was, possibly more. When Maryanne and I had gotten married, he was still in middle school. He held a cup of beer in one hand and a cigarette in the other. He grinned and I spotted a few missing teeth.

"Holy shit," I said. "Matt?"

He looked exactly like his biological father and namesake, Mattie, whom Maryanne and I would occasionally visit when we were still together. Mattie was an alcoholic who lived in a small room in a dodgy part of Harrisburg, where he eventually drank himself to death.

I found Holly and stood by her side for the rest of the afternoon. Something about meeting Matt had put me in a somber mood. The kids played. We ate. None of us had ever seen a roast hog before and it was a sight, splayed out on a folding table, head and snout still attached. Before we left, I congratulated Joey again. The next time I saw him was at the ceremony, wearing his cap and gown.

I had never been to a high-school graduation before. I felt so proud as I watched Joey in his cap and gown. He held his head high and grinned. He pumped his fist to some of his classmates and they pumped their fists back.

The day before we were to leave for Seattle, I drove over to Maryanne's house by myself in the rental car. I thought I'd give the amends thing another shot.

I rang the bell and Maryanne answered. "Joey's not here," she said.

"I know," I said. Joey had gone to the Maryland beaches with his friends. "I wanted to talk with you."

"Okay," she said. Maryanne put her fist on her hip. "What's up?"

She looked right into my face. Maryanne is a very direct woman who always says what's on her mind. My mouth dried up. Cars rushed past on Route 322.

"Out here," I said.

"You want to come in?" she asked.

She stepped back from the door and motioned with her head. I thought I heard just a hint of irritation in her voice. She held a dishrag in her hand.

I wiped my feet and came into the house.

Jack was sitting in the living room watching TV. Maryanne had stopped just past Jack and then turned to face me. Jack greeted me and Maryanne announced to the room at large that I had something I wanted to tell her.

Jack nodded but kept watching his football game. I wished I had stayed out on the porch. I started to grin so big my cheeks began to ache.

"Tim," Maryanne said. "You're grinning like a fool. What's on your mind?"

"Well . . ." I said.

What had I come here to say? I had no idea. I hadn't really prepared remarks. I had assumed the right words would just come to me. Maryanne furrowed her brow. I looked at the dishrag in her hand wondered what task I was keeping her from. Jack stopped looking at the TV and glanced up at me.

"I guess this means I can stop paying child support." I said.

I may have meant it as a joke. Or maybe an ironic comment. To be honest, I was a little surprised to hear it, as if it had come from someone else's mouth. As soon as I said it, though, I knew it was all wrong.

Maryanne's mouth fell open. Jack averted his eyes, putting his hand up to cover his face. He may have snorted, but I couldn't be sure. My forehead had become wet and my shirt felt clammy under my arms.

Maryanne's face went bright red. She started to lecture me about how hard it was to raise a child. How expensive everything was. Her finger wagged, she leaned forward.

I licked my lips and held my arms. I felt like such an ass. The whole idea with making amends was not to further injure the person you were making amends with. Sort of like the doctors' oath, "*First do no harm.*" Maryanne was totally pissed off, ranting. I was totally fucking it up. Again. What could I do? I stood silently and waited for Maryanne to stop.

"And what about those braces," Maryanne said. Joey had needed braces near the start of middle school. "Those braces cost five thousand dollars. I paid five thousand dollars. Five. Thousand. Dollars."

"And you got a million-dollar smile," Jack said. He was grinning. He stretched opened his arms and held his hands palm up. "Seems like a good deal to me," he said.

Maryanne stopped and looked at her husband.

I felt so grateful for Jack.

"I should probably go," I said.

Maryanne stalked out of the room.

"Okay, Tim," Jack said. He had already gone back to watching the game. "We'll see you around."

* * *

Joey earned a football scholarship. He was headed to a small Pennsylvania school near the New York State line. He told me the name of the school, but I wasn't familiar with it. He described some of the technicalities of the scholarship, but it was mostly a sports thing and didn't make much sense to me. Nevertheless, I was pleased for him.

He left for football camp in the hottest part of the summer.

Just as the days were beginning to get shorter and darker, the phone rang at our home in Seattle. It was Joey. "You're going to be mad," he said.

He had left campus. He didn't like being away from home, didn't care for the academic rigor of college. The new plan was to find a job and live with Maryanne and Jack. They had moved back into the small house in the Zoo. He was back in Steelton.

I felt disappointed, but I tried not to linger on those feelings. I reminded myself that everyone had to find his or her own path.

"I loved college," I said, "but it might not be right for you—*yet.*"

Joey seemed disappointed with himself.

I reminded him that he was a high school graduate, which was a much better outcome than I had ever managed. "When I was your age," I said, "I had been shooting heroin for almost a year. Compared to me, you're batting a thousand."

Joey got a job delivering sheetrock with one of Maryanne's younger brothers. Joey loved his uncles. I continued to call. Occasionally when we talked, he would tell me things that made little sense. Once he complained that he had hurt the knuckles on both his hands.

"Were you fighting?" I asked.

"Nope," Joey said.

I pressed him, but he said he couldn't remember how his hands had been hurt.

"Maybe it happened at work," he said.

"Yeah," I said. "Maybe you slammed the door on both your hands?"

I chuckled.

He didn't laugh.

"Were you drinking?" I asked. My voice went flat.

I would eventually learn that this question, coming from me in that flat monotone, could immediately shut down any conversation Joey and I were having. *Were you drinking, son?* It's your recovering alcoholic, reformed heroin-addict father calling to ask if you were drinking. *Were you having any fun, son?* Over the years, in recovery meetings, I had heard many fathers lament their sons' behavior. Often you never heard the child's side of the story. I always wondered if those fathers were projecting their own poor drinking habits onto their boys. One thing was for sure—those nagging fathers never seemed to draw much closer to their sons.

I didn't want to turn into a nag. In recovery programs, the conventional wisdom is that fathers make lousy sponsors for their sons anyway. But if I'd make a crappy sponsor, I resolved to be the best father I could. I decided to watch and wait.

Occasionally when I spoke to my younger brother, a Steelton police officer, he would try to describe events that he thought I ought to know about. One time he told me about a disturbance that involved Joey. The police call had come in a few weeks before, and my brother had waited to tell me about it. He hadn't responded to the call, but he knew the officer who had.

"A disturbance?" I repeated the word.

"Joey was there," my brother said. "Along with some other boys."

"What happened?" I asked.

"Someone's truck was damaged," my brother said.

"A car accident?" I asked.

"Not exactly," he said. "But it was about $400 in damages."

"How did it get damaged?" I asked.

"I don't know. I wasn't there," he said. "Maybe someone punched it."

"Punched the truck?" I asked. I was surprised.

"Yep," he said. "$400 dollars in punches."

That just seemed crazy to me. Who punches a truck? I did what any good father would do. I defended my son: "What are you trying to say here?" I asked. "My Joey is a good boy."

* * *

Two years after Joey graduated, I planned another trip to Pennsylvania. Joey and his friends had purchased a small trailer on the Susquehanna River, where they spent most of their time doing whatever it is young men do on riverbanks. I wasn't sure there was anything I could do to entice him to hang out with me and my seven-year-olds on our visit. Holly suggested a weekend trip to Manhattan.

"The Big Apple?" Joey said. I could hear surprise and delight in his voice. "I'll go to the city with you guys."

We visited with my family for a few days and then met up with Joey. We all boarded a train into Manhattan for the Fourth of July weekend. On the train ride into the city, Amtrak delayed the train just before we hit Pennsylvania Station. I reminded Joey about all the times I would invite him to my apartment in the Bronx, but he always declined, saying he was too scared to go to New York.

"I was just little," Joey said.

He sounded defensive, but he smiled and looked out the window. I hadn't intended to put him on guard.

"To be honest," I said, "I was probably more scared than you were."

"What did you have to be scared about?" he asked. He twisted in his seat to look at my face.

"Oh, son. . ." I said. I grinned and shook my head.

There was a beat of silence.

"You," I said. "My ability to take care of you—everything."

There was a certain hunger in the look he gave me that I hadn't seen in many years. "You probably sensed my fear," I said, "even if you didn't know it. Kids are smart." I glanced at my twins in the seat across the aisle.

The train started rolling.

We took a rollicking cab ride from Pennsylvania Station to an apartment, loaned to us by a friend in the East Village, where we were to stay that weekend. I was excited to be back in the city. While Holly took the twins to get something to eat, Joey and I went into the night.

Joey seemed energized by the crowds, the wide, flat rivers of sidewalk, even the lights and the sounds of traffic. I led us to Saint Mark's Place and stopped in the middle of the block.

"Hold on, son," I said. "Hold on."

I felt emboldened by our conversation on the train. I wanted to show Joey the homeless shelter where I stayed my first few weeks in the city, but I couldn't find it. I spotted Trash and Vaudeville, a boutique clothing store I remembered for its unusual name and storefront with mannequins dressed in black leather and lace. Using the store as a reference, I found an unfamiliar brick building with retail stores at street level on the north side of the block where the shelter had once stood.

The shelter had been torn down: The Electric Circus was no more.

"When I first came to New York, there was a homeless shelter over there," I said. "I stayed there until I got into treatment."

"You were homeless?" Joey said. "In a shelter?"

I chuckled at the shock in his voice.

"We were always so hungry," I said, "I remember my first night; this big black lady took pity on me and shared some macaroni she had boiled up."

We were standing on the curb, letting the crowds of young people swarm past us.

"She put this huge dump of macaroni on a paper plate," I said. I used my hands to show how big. "You know what I told her?"

Joey tilted his head.

"I said, 'What—no tomato sauce?'" I grinned.

Joey raised his eyebrow. "That's what you told her?" he asked.

"You ever eat macaronis with no tomato sauce?" I said.

We laughed and started walking.

We ended up in Washington Square Park, where we grabbed a bench on the periphery of the park under a pool of light from a nearby streetlamp. Drug dealers hawked product in the mostly deserted park; some things never change. Nevertheless, I felt so pleased with this trip, I seemed to be finally finding my groove with my oldest boy. Joey was telling me something about his new security job with the county, and his larger plans to pursue a career in law enforcement.

"I'm going to join the military," Joey said.

"Wait—what?" I said.

The United States had troops deployed in Afghanistan. We had just invaded Iraq. I thought it was a terrible idea. I decided to finally weigh in, to offer an opinion, to use my influence as a parent to guide my child in a different direction, a direction I felt might offer him a more promising future. I had been watching and waiting for years now and that *had* seemed like a good strategy. But this was a terrible idea. Somebody could get hurt.

There was a time to act and the time was now!

I tried to talk him out of it. I arranged with Holly for our family to lend him money to attend the local police academy. I got my younger brother to agree to put Joey up at his house during his time at the academy. But all my maneuvering proved useless.

Joey had already decided. He was diplomatic, but firm. His mind was made up. Nothing I said could convince him otherwise. As I struggled to come to terms with his decision, I remembered having had almost the exact same conversation with my father about joining the military. Dad said I'd end up getting my head shot off; I'd said he was being dramatic.

In so many ways, Joey was completely different from me. But in other ways I saw an eerie similarity.

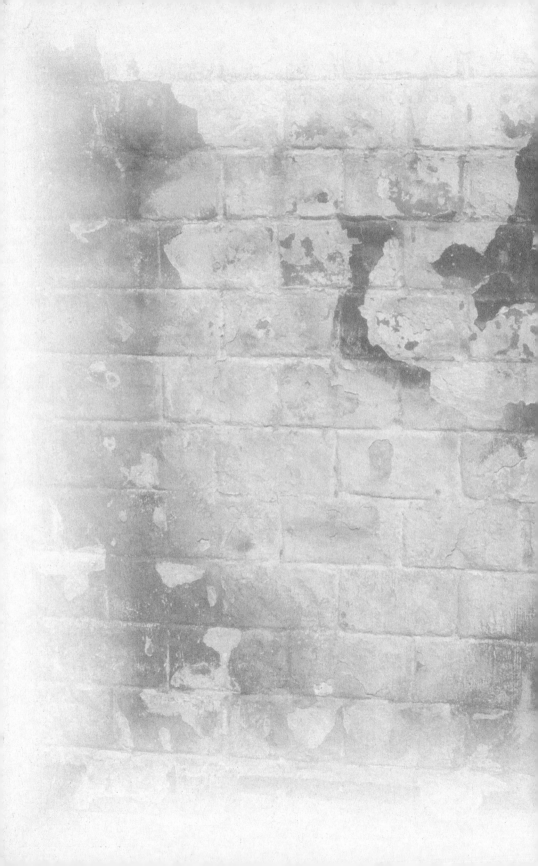

CHAPTER 11

SPIRITUAL AWARENESS

Joey finished Coast Guard boot camp and Port Seattle was his first assignment. We hadn't lived in the same city since he was three years old. When he told me, I couldn't believe my good fortune. Holly and I were about to move our eight-year-old twins into separate rooms, but instead we let them share a little longer. I moved my computer out of the small bedroom to make room for Joey.

Almost immediately, Maryanne reached out to offer me parenting tips.

She told me that Joey needed more food than I might realize but he felt embarrassed by how much he ate and probably wouldn't ask for seconds. "If you go to McDonalds," she said, "you have to get him at least three Big Macs." We had never before had discussions about Joey's specific needs, and I felt delighted that she was willing to bring me into her confidence. I could hear the anxiety in her voice. For both their lives, this was the first time Joey had been more than an overnight car ride away from her care. I felt needed. I would be participating in Joey's life in a way that was new to all of us.

The kids and I picked up Joey at the airport.

He had always worn his hair clipped short, but he looked different in his uniform: He seemed sharper, more mature, and even a little aloof. On Sunday, I invited Joey to attend church with our family. I made the suggestion sheepishly, prepared for him to beg off, but he surprised me by readily accepting.

When it came to spirituality and church, I felt fortunate that Holly and I were both in recovery. Neither of us was big on religion, but we both felt a certain responsibility to set a spiritual cadence for our family, especially when the twins were small. Neither of us used a strictly religious rudder to guide our family's ship, and we often ended up improvising with a spiritual mash-up of twelve-step principles and Catholicism. It didn't always work out the way we expected. One morning, Holly had been getting the kids ready for school as she usually did. She was upset about something and we were discussing it discreetly as we got the kids' lunches packed and backpacks loaded.

The kids were already in the car. I had been listening and nodding all morning long, practicing my best twelve-step form. Holly and I stood at the door of the house.

"That sounds like a challenging situation," I said. "What do you think your Higher Power is trying to tell you?"

Holly slowly turned, looked into my face and scowled.

I had to work to suppress my grin. She and I were cut from the same cloth. When Roger used to tell me this sort of thing on the telephone, I would roll my eyes and think: "Oh, *fuck you* very much." But I'd always found relief from my problems this way, and I hoped she would, too.

Holly got into the car.

I waved good-bye from the porch.

The kids waved from the backseat.

Holly rolled down her window and put her arm out. She raised her hand over the roof so the kids couldn't see, and then she flipped me the bird.

I grinned and gave her the thumbs up. We only had to shoot for spiritual progress, not perfection. I felt comfortable with the spiritual landscape of my new life, but I felt less certain of myself when it came to sharing it with Joey. How would it all appear to him?

He didn't balk about going to church when I asked him; however, he reminded me that he had gone to church with my mother when he was younger. I told him we were going to a Catholic church. Maryanne had sent him to Catholic elementary school, so I knew he was familiar with the service.

St. Therese was an unconventional mix of Catholic and Baptist traditions. Holly and I loved the blended congregation of white, black, straight, and gay, as well as the gospel choir that belted out songs during the sacrament. When we'd first gone searching for churches, we'd come to St. Therese because Holly had heard their gospel choir. I was just looking for someplace that felt right. We'd sat in the balcony, and I spotted a white-haired deacon below who looked familiar. This man turned out to be none other than Dave, my first sponsor in Seattle. I hadn't seen him in years! After the kids were born, I had stopped calling. We met after the service and Dave seemed delighted. He told me that his sponsor (my grand-sponsor) was Father Nicholas, one of the priests.

I knew this was the right church for us.

Father Nicholas had a rugged face, gentle eyes, and an easygoing disposition. His homilies were always a wonderful mixture of scripture, twelve-step recovery, and sage humor. His examination of scripture through the prism of the principles of recovery made the verses come alive for me.

Once, I'd been sitting in the pew listening to Father Nicholas's homily. He was just getting over a cold and you could hear it in his voice. My then seven-year-old son tugged on my shirt sleeve. I tried to wave him off, but he wanted to tell me something.

I leaned down and put my ear near his mouth.

"Jesus's voice sounds much better this week," he said.

I was amused and filled with a sense of surprise and awe. I resisted the urge to correct him. My child was grappling with one of the biggest mysteries of faith: Who is God? I was pleased he had an answer. I figured he'd reevaluate throughout his life.

I know I certainly had.

"His voice does sound better," I said.

I once went to see Father Nicholas when the self-loathing for moving so far from Joey became too difficult to bear. We'd had a Saturday afternoon appointment, and I'd laid out the whole situation for him. Father Nicholas listened. When I finished, he finally spoke. "I hate to tell you," he said, "but you're a *mensch*."

I felt terrible, but snorted at his use of Yiddish.

"Seriously," he said. "There is nothing here to forgive."

So it was with much pride and a little trepidation that I escorted Joey through the great doors of the church that Sunday morning in the brisk fall air, with the bright morning sun at our backs. Father Nicholas was in the doorway, greeting the congregation. As I approached, I saw Father Nicholas's eyes sweep from my face to a point up and beyond my right shoulder.

I introduced Joey.

Joey stepped up. He squared his shoulders and thrust out his hand.

"Good morning, sir," he said.

He offered small talk about his experience in the Seattle area and the military. He may have even complimented Father Nicholas on the appearance of the church, which was decorated with school children's drawings for Thanksgiving.

I stood in the entry of the church and beamed.

One weekend, I drove Joey to the base for duty. He looked sharp in his working uniform, with a duffle bag on his lap. But I wondered if he were beginning to regret having signed up. Shortly after I enlisted, I realized that the service wasn't right for me. I felt trapped and terrible, with almost an entire four-year enlistment stretching out before me.

"What do you think of the military so far, son?" I asked.

"Dad," Joey said. His voice sounded so grave, I turned to look at his face. His chin was set, he was serious. "I love it," he said. "I love waking up in the morning. I love going to work on the boat. This is absolutely the best job I have ever had."

I hadn't expected to hear such conviction.

The structure and discipline of military life had made him blossom. Soon the accolades started to roll in: positive reviews from his superiors and peers, a promotion to seaman, and then Sailor of the Quarter two consecutive quarters running. He thrived in the military in a way I had never been able to. I began to wonder if the nagging voice at the back of my mind about his drinking were really just a projection of my own behavior.

One day Joey told me he didn't want to go to church with us on Sundays anymore.

I was disappointed but accepted it. I remembered how my mother had always insisted I attend church with her when I was still using drugs and needed money or a place to stay. She'd drive us to the church in her car, and I always seemed to forget about the altar call until we got to that part of the service. The pastor would call all the sinners in the congregation to the altar and Mom would give me a withering look. I'd sigh. I had no choice but to trek down to the front of the church and let the pastor lay hands on me to pray.

I didn't want to do Joey that way.

I knew of a recovery speaker-meeting on Saturday nights that was popular with the young people. I signed up to speak and invited Joey to tag along. The meeting was held in a church basement. We got there and found a small crowd of smokers standing outside the door. We hustled inside to a tightly packed room, alive with loud conversation, laughter, and the smell of fresh-brewed coffee. Joey was standing at my elbow and looked around the room. Young, tattooed men stood around in baggy pants and baseball caps, drinking coffee. Girls milled about in groups of two or three. Most of these young ladies wore tight jeans, thick belts, and clingy shirts that crept up their tummies. Some had bellybutton rings glittering in their navels. Others had little tattoos, peeking out of the waist bands of their pants.

"What do you think?" I asked.

Joey grinned.

"This is alright," he said.

I felt pleased. I had found a spiritual community Joey and I could both live with.

* * *

Holly and I planned a trip to LA. Holly had signed up for a weekend writing conference. We were going to vacation and visit her brother and father who lived in Redondo Beach for a few days. Then we would descend on the hotel for our final weekend at the conference. I asked Joey if he wanted to join us. He made arrangements to take a few days off at the tail end of our trip. We made plans to fly him down for the weekend to meet up with us.

We checked into our hotel Thursday morning and I was splayed out on the bed. Joey would fly in the next morning. I was looking forward to exploring LA with him, just like we had done in Manhattan. My phone rang and I saw Joey's number appear in the caller ID window.

I felt mild apprehension. He had warned me he might get a last minute assignment.

"Joe?" I said. "We just checked into the hotel and it's sweet."

I knew my voice sounded far too cheerful, but I couldn't help it. I was bracing myself for bad news. "I think you're going to like it," I said.

"Hey Pop," Joey said. He voice sounded sullen. "That's great."

"What's up son?" I asked. "Do you have to cancel? Did something come up?" I hadn't meant to voice my fears, but his voice sounded so weighted, the words had slipped out of my mouth before I could stop them.

"No, no, no," he said. "I'm still coming." He answered quickly, probably in response to the disappointment he heard in my voice.

I felt confused. There was a beat of silence.

"I mean," Joey said, "if you still want me to come."

Another beat of silence.

I sat up on the bed and held the phone to my ear.

"Look, I wrecked your car," Joey said. "Last night."

I asked if anyone was hurt, although I was already pretty certain no one was. "No injuries," he said. I asked how bad. "Pretty bad," he said. But you could still drive it. It had happened as he was parking the car. No other cars involved.

"Were you drinking?" I asked.

Joey sighed.

"Dad," he said. I could hear impatience in his voice.

"Yes, I was drinking," he said. "But that didn't have anything to do with it."

I snorted. "Son," I said. "Nothing?"

I was disappointed and wanted to get off the phone. I asked him to tell Holly what he had just told me and handed her the phone. Holly listened, then told him not to worry. "Accidents happen to everyone," she said.

I was so impressed with how Holly responded. She was caring and nurturing, just like every good sponsor I had ever had had been. I decided to take my lead from her. I motioned that I wanted to talk again. She finished and handed the phone to me.

I said I was glad he wasn't hurt. I pointed out how fortunate we were no other cars were involved and that we could still drive the Jetta. Once I started articulating all we had to be grateful for, my anger began to slip away. My enthusiasm for our trip quickly returned. I encouraged him to get on the plane the next day and listed all the things we could do together in LA. As I spoke, I felt more and more certain that I had chosen the right tack. It wouldn't do us any good to let a car accident come between us, no matter the circumstances. One time on leave from the Navy, I'd had a driving accident in my mother's Hornet that had torn a great hole in one of the fenders—and then had left her and my brothers to deal with the repairs. I remembered how terrible I felt. I told Joey he could pay for the deductible of the repair and we'd be straight on the car.

He said he would.

If nothing else, I realized that one good thing had come of this event; I understood now that not all of Joey's problems with alcohol were solely in my imagination.

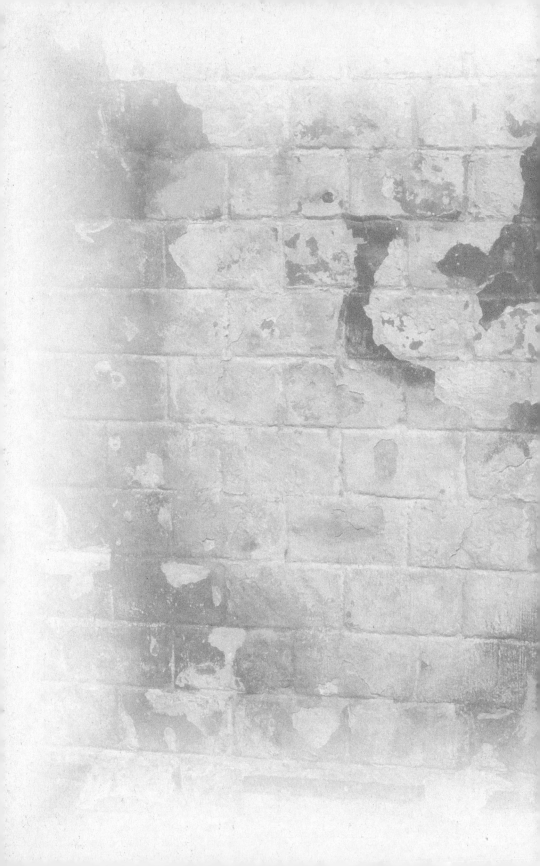

CHAPTER 12

SERVICE

After a year, the Coast Guard reassigned Joey to Port Miami.

I was sad. I moped. I changed teams at work. On the new team, we had an upcoming product release that would coincide with the holidays. To carve out a place for myself on the new team, I threw myself into the job. I wanted to ensure that my part in the release was a complete success. Joey called as he settled into his new life in Miami. We discussed the challenges of starting over at work—he at a new duty station, me on a new product team. He had been promoted to Petty Officer Third Class and was already studying for the exam for the next pay grade. I felt much closer to him than ever before, but our conversations were mostly about our jobs.

One morning Joey called as I was walking our dog.

"I have to tell you something," he said. His voice sounded grave. I stood and let the dog tug at his leash. "I got a DUI last night," he said.

"Driving under the influence?" I asked.

"Yep," Joey said, "affirmative."

The civilian police officer who had pulled him over had handed him off to the military authorities on base for discipline. He wasn't sure if he'd be able to remain in the military. He sounded mortified. In the last twenty years, the consequences for DUI have changed dramatically, but even I was surprised that his enlistment was on the line. I told him how in the recovery meetings you would often hear the old guys talk about getting DUIs and only paying fines to keep their driver's license. "But now," I said, "it's a whole new ball game."

Joey sounded despondent.

I encouraged him to find out more about what his options were. Even as I asked him to explore his own options, I agonized about what my own might be. How should I respond to these developments? The conventional wisdom that fathers made lousy sponsors seemed borne out by my own experience; my biggest gains with Joey seemed to have come by minding my own business, remaining detached. It never worked for me to weigh in on the obvious, like how much he drank or his occasional run-in with authorities. My role, it seemed, was to be supportive, provide a little cash, and revel in his accomplishments. Of course, this was easier to do if I allowed myself to believe there were no recovery issues to worry about. For me, the hardest part of being a good father was resisting the urge to become a nag. In the meantime, I had to trust that Joey would learn from his own experiences and that the lessons wouldn't be too difficult for either of us to bear.

As the drama played out, I discovered that Joey would be remanded to outpatient treatment at the VA. Based on his treatment outcome, he might be able to keep his enlistment, but he would certainly lose his rank.

Joey was disappointed about the rank, but he seemed resigned to save his enlistment.

I encouraged him to do just that.

Over the next few days, he began calling me more. He called one weekend, and I was in the office, working toward a deadline. I saw his name appear in the caller ID window and decided to take a break. I asked how he was making out and then put my feet up on the desk. These days, Joey had plenty to say.

As we talked, he asked for my opinion on something. One thing I had learned as a non-custodial parent was to always ask for context before offering an opinion. This way I could offer my view without saying anything I'd later regret.

"What does your mom say?" I asked.

"To be honest," Joey said, "I couldn't tell you." His voice was heavy. "We haven't spoken much the last few days."

"Why not?" I asked. Joey and Maryanne usually spoke with one another every day, sometimes more than once a day.

Joey hesitated. He started to say he didn't know, but I cut him off.

"—because of the DUI charges?" I asked.

He sighed. There was a beat of silence.

"I guess," he said. His voice was low. "She's upset with me."

A great wave of empathy washed over me. I could hear the shame in his voice. I knew what it felt like to screw up so bad your own mother wouldn't speak to you.

I put my feet on the floor. I had to swallow to find my voice.

"I know how you feel, son," I said.

I got up. Stretching out the cord on my phone to its limits, I kicked the door to my office shut. I stood by my desk with my hand in my pocket, the phone to my ear.

"One time," I said. "This was back when you were little—"

"I went to your gram's house. The front door was locked, and back then we never locked our door. So I knocked. I peeked in the living room window but couldn't see anything. It was October, I was cold. My mom's car was in the lot, but I couldn't be sure if anyone was home. All of a sudden, the Steelton police rolled up, lights flashing."

"What—" Joey said. I had his attention.

"You know Pickles?" I asked. Pickles was Officer Callahan, a wiry black man who had been on the force since I was a boy. He owned an automotive garage in Steelton and had been a guest at my brother's wedding.

"Everybody knows Pickles," Joey said.

"Pickles got out of the cruiser and told me I had to leave. But I didn't understand what was happening. I was cold and annoyed that the door was locked, so I ignored Pickles and knocked on the door again."

"Gram called the cops?" Joey asked.

"She did," I said. "Joey, if a cop ever asks you to do something, my advice to you is to do it. Pickles came up on the porch, and he did some shit to my arms—"

Joey gasped; I laughed.

"Son, it was terrible. I thought my arm was going to come off."

"I know that move," Joey said. "We study it for law enforcement drills."

I chuckled.

There was a short pause, and neither of us said anything.

"My mom came out on the porch. By then I had figured out that she had called the cops, so I started yelling at her—"

Joey blew air out of his mouth.

"—And she didn't like what Pickles was doing to my arms, so she started yelling at Pickles—"

Joey chuckled. "Go, Gram."

"—All the neighbors came out. The police lights were going. All the people in the Zoo were on their porches."

"Holy shit," Joey said. "I didn't know any of this."

"Yeah," I said. "It was terrible."

"You know how it ended?" I asked. "Pickles whispered, 'Don't make me kick your ass in front of your mom.'" I laughed. "Fucking Pickles."

Joey laughed.

He made a low, whistling noise.

"But you and Gram are cool now, right?" he asked.

"We are," I said. "But it took time. In fact, your mom was the one who got me and my mom back together for our first conversation after the thing with Pickles."

We started to talk about disappointing our mothers.

"It's not so bad that you disappoint your mom," I said. "God knows I still do things that disappoint my mom. What felt horrible was realizing that my mom didn't have a choice. I put her in a terrible position."

We started talking about treatment. Joey said his was twelve weeks long, and he didn't know how he would make it. I said mine had lasted eighteen months, then savored Joey's shocked response.

As we spoke, I thought about the idea that fathers made lousy sponsors. But my intuition told me I was on the right track, saying the right things. I had waited in the wings for years and now I was up; it was showtime.

An unconventional paternal relationship with Joey—the very thing that had caused me such grief and pain over the years—might be my greatest asset. No one else in his family or mine was in recovery. There were no role models here. All I had was a vague recollection of the Crazy Aunt archetype my writer teacher Tess Gallant had mentioned many years ago in college, and a burning desire to love my son. If my job was to sweep in from afar and offer a perspective the boy might otherwise not ever have considered, I was damn well going to put on the petticoats and get the job done. This conversation might be the very reason why God had put me on the planet. Who else was going to do it? I am Joey's father.

We talked for hours.

When we finished, Joey seemed enthusiastic. I was thrilled. I told him he could call me back the next day or even sooner if he wanted. I told him what my sponsor had always told me—call me whenever you want to or need to. I was available to talk.

* * *

I took calls from Joey every day over the next few weeks.

I trotted out all the things my sponsor had ever said to me. One time Joey told me he got a parking ticket, and I immediately said, 'I'm really glad to hear that!' just like Roger would have said to me when I reported some mundane tragedy.

"You're glad?" Joey said. I could hear the irritation in his voice.

"Absolutely, son." I said.

This was the part where Roger would whip out some fancy reasoning that explained why what had just happened was actually "not that bad," and perhaps even the "best possible outcome."

I felt mild panic.

And then I found myself explaining that during treatment it was good to run into a little adversity. "Treatment is probably the only time in your life when you will be surrounded by professionals all geared to offer you support. If no challenges come up, you might not learn anything."

I didn't know where that explanation had come from, but it sounded reasonable to me. And no one was more surprised than me that it had actually come out of my mouth.

"You know what cops always say about recovering addicts?" I asked. "'As soon as he breaks a shoelace, he'll be back on the shit.'" I laughed. "Fucking cops, right?—"

"But there's some truth in there," I said. "Addicts and alcoholics cope with life by using drugs and alcohol. Part of your job in treatment is to find new ways to cope."

"It's a fifty-dollar ticket," Joey said.

I chuckled. "Money well spent, son. Money well spent."

By the time we got off the phone, we both saw the bigger picture. And I was amazed at how well I seemed to be doing. Joey seemed enthused. I remembered getting off the phone with Roger and feeling the same way. I was delighted.

One afternoon Joey called with something he couldn't quite put into words.

"The group counseling at the VA," Joey said, "is strange."

"How so?" I asked.

"I don't want to sound racist or anything," Joey said, "but it's all old black men from Vietnam. I'm the youngest, whitest person in the group."

I laughed, remembering my experience at Rockford. I hadn't thought about Blackman or Terrance Tyson in years. What sweet friends to have had.

"Mine had five hundred teenage crack heads from all five New York City boroughs," I said. "You have to trust that God has you in the right place. You find yourself in an uncomfortable position—well, maybe that means you need a little experience being uncomfortable." I was already thinking ahead to Joey's first leave after treatment. I wasn't even sure what his plans were once treatment had ended. Would he resume social drinking after his restrictions were lifted?

I asked, and he said he was done. His intention was to remain in recovery. Joey didn't want any more grief.

"When you go home," I said, "you're going to be the only one who isn't drinking."

The phone went quiet. Standing alone on something like social drinking could be one of the hardest things a person could do with their family and friends.

"I'm not down with all the Higher Power stuff," Joey said, changing the subject.

I laughed. "That's okay."

"If you believe in a Higher Power," Joey asked, "then do you feel like everything will, what—work itself out?"

"Well, no—" I said. "Bad shit happens every day. Everything changes when you begin recovery, but that's one thing that remains the same. Bad shit will continue to happen."

Joey laughed.

"But I believe if I do everything in my power to keep my life on track, then if some bad shit does happen, I won't have anything to be ashamed of. And, hopefully, I'll be in a better shape—emotionally, intellectually, and spiritually—to deal with it, whatever it is."

I had never had much luck with new guys in the program, but I poured it all into these phone calls. As the holidays got closer, my work got even more crazy and affected. Everyone needed something from me. To deal with the stress, I went back to basics myself. When I felt panicky about whether I would have enough time to meet my obligations, I told myself "One Day at a Time." If I had an important meeting and my son called, I thought "First Things First," and asked if I could call him back.

Holly started pestering me to get the Christmas lights up. I had been waiting for a break in the weather since Thanksgiving, but every day it rained and rained. One morning on my way out the door, Holly said "Lights?" and I sighed. There was a misting rain, but it was less than two weeks before Christmas. I got the ladder and spent the next two hours attaching multicolored lights to the trim of our small ranch house. When I finished, my hair was damp and my fingers were numb. I had about half an hour to make a meeting at work.

Feeling miserable, I drove to campus.

Later that day, Joey called, and he sounded morose.

"This is going to be a terrible Christmas," he said.

I had to agree that Christmas in treatment was depressing. We started to talk about feeling depressed. I started thinking about how much my life had changed since the year I spent Christmas in treatment.

"Maybe this is your terrible Christmas," I said.

"Maybe one Christmas," I said, "in the not too distant future, you might have a wife and some kids. And maybe your wife will be grousing at you to get the Christmas lights up. Maybe it will be raining, and you'll have a ton of work to get done at your job. And you'll think: '*This is the worst Christmas there could ever be!*'"

"But then you'll think—No, wait. There was that one Christmas I spent in treatment." I laughed. "Never hurts to have a terrible Christmas in your back pocket, son."

Joey told me how he longed to have a family of his own. We talked about how good it felt to belong. When I got off the phone, I hoped Joey felt better. But what felt remarkable to me was how much my own outlook had improved. When I drove up to my home later that night, I shut off my car and sat listening to the engine tick, watching the little lights I had strung that morning glitter in the dark night.

Somehow we all got through the holidays.

I did my part at work and we shipped our new product. I did my part at home and we enjoyed Christmas. One day Joey called and told me he had been speaking to his mother. When I learned that he had begun to repair his relationship with Maryanne, I felt certain he was going to make it. Joey told me that he mentioned to his mother what had been happening with our relationship. I realized that we had changed in some subtle, but powerful ways. He recognized it and so did I.

But I still had not made amends to Maryanne.

I have never heard of anyone emailing an amend to their ex-wife, but that was exactly what I did. I took responsibility for our disastrous marriage, for my selfish behavior, and for my overwhelming needs, which almost sank us all. I asked her what I could do to make it right.

After I hit send, I felt foolish. Who emails amends?

For weeks I heard nothing. I had almost forgotten about it.

And then, finally, I got this short reply:

"Don't sweat it, Tim. I had my own demons to slay."

And just like that, I had made my amends.

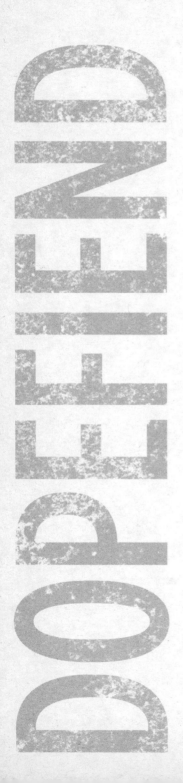

EPILOGUE

I wrote this story in about six months. For years, I had been struggling to write a different book, a memoir about the relationship I had with my own father, but I could never quite wrap my mind around how the narrative ought to work. This is probably because I still don't quite know what to do with the relationship I had with my father. He died when I was eighteen. He wasn't an easy man to know. He was kind, politically progressive, even spiritual in his own way. But he kept to himself. He had an explosive temper. I remember mostly how deeply I longed to know him. As it turns out, even that much longing isn't enough to write a book. I finally had to give up. Had to set that story aside. What to do next?

When the idea to write about recovery came to mind, I knew almost immediately the story would have to be about my relationship with Joey. There was just no other way to tell it. My relationship with Joey pushed me into recovery in the first place. Over the years, my role as a non-custodial parent has been one of the single driving beats, a consistent hum and certain, constant rhythm to my life. True, I have met and fallen in love with a beautiful woman. She is now my best friend, and we have created two glorious children together. This, of course, is all wonderful. I am grateful to have such a rich life. But when I think of my own net worth as a person, the calculations always seem to come round to my relationship with Joey. And this is probably only because I have thought so long and critically about my own father's performance as a parent. In light of my experience with fatherhood, I have had to make some necessary adjustments, both on my side of the ledger and on his.

All of this reckoning only amplifies for me that paternal relationships have a long-lasting but mutable quality. Stories may come to a satisfying and redemptive close, but fathers and sons will continue to examine and judge one another, sometimes even long after one or the other has gone to the grave. This seems necessary and appropriate. I know I relate to my father much differently today than I did when I was eighteen. No one can know how they'll make out in such calculations. And this, too, seems appropriate and fine to me. I did not write this to defend my abilities as a parent or father. I wrote it because fatherhood is important to me. And, of course, because I feel it's a good story that deserves to be told.

And what about recovery?

Consider the following: I am pretty sure that all of my past police records have been expunged. Although I took advantage of a variety of drug treatment facilities, I would be very surprised if there were actually any records of my experience, in any facility. Drug treatment services come and go. They often operate on shoestring budgets, and I used them just as digital record keeping was becoming the standard. Meanwhile, at the other end of the records-keeping spectrum, I graduated *summa cum laude* from Hunter College. I've earned a number of professional certificates, including the Microsoft Certified Systems Engineer (MCSE) certification. And if we're willing to forgo official records and consider hearsay evidence, I haven't shot up any fucking heroin in more than twenty years.

I mean, *come on.*

The question about recovery, then, becomes this: Why go on and on about it? Why not just *move on*, for God's sake? How long must one remain abstinent? If there exist no official records of failure and only official records of success, where is the wisdom in continuing to call oneself an addict? There is a strong social stigma associated with the word addict. Should we continue to label ourselves this way? I think like this from time to time. I can't help it. My mind is open and expansive and questioning and it wanders the paths on which it wants to tread. But then I get a phone call, and in the caller ID window I see Joey's name. Or I see a picture of Joey's lovely wife on a social-networking website, or one of his new baby daughters, my gorgeous little granddaughters.

And I think, "Well, okay—one more day won't hurt.

"After all, it's just one day."

* * *

When I finally made my last support payment here in Seattle, I called the child support office and spoke to my caseworker. She was a kind woman. Without her help, I would have never been able to sort through certain logistical issues and purchase my home. She noted with delight that my final payment was at hand and offered me, unsolicited, a tally of all the support I had paid over the years. I could hear her tapping away at her keyboard.

Finally she said, "Well, I usually tell you guys, 'You could have bought a house for what you spent on this child.' But you—," she paused. "You haven't accumulated enough to have purchased a house. You could have bought—"she paused again.

"—a car," she said.

I knew she was a nice woman and that she didn't mean me any harm. I may have even chuckled politely, the habit being so strong.

"—a small car," she added.

Some might think that I got off easy with paying my debts, but they would be wrong. One way or another, you pay for everything in this life. No matter what you do, nothing is free.

Nothing except the grace of God.

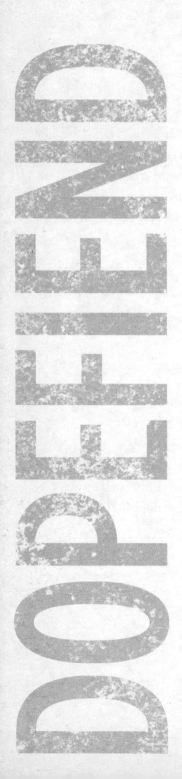

Of Character: Building Assets in Recovery
Denise D. Crosson, Ph.D. • $12.95 US • ISBN-13: 978-0-9799869-2-5

RELATIONSHIPS

From Heartbreak to Heart's Desire: Developing a Healthy GPS (Guy Picking System)
Dawn Maslar, MS • $14.95 US • ISBN-13: 978-0-9818482-6-6

Disentangle: When You've Lost Your Self in Someone Else
Nancy L. Johnston, MS, LPC, LSATP • $15.95 US
ISBN-13: 978-1-936290-03-1

YOUNG ADULT AND YOUNG READER

First Star I See
Jaye Andras Caffrey, illustrated by Lynne Adamson • $12.95 US
ISBN-13: 978-1-936290-01-7

The Secret of Willow Ridge: Gabe's Dad Finds Recovery
Helen H. Moore, illustrated by John Blackford
Foreword by Claudia Black, Ph.D. • $12.95 US
ISBN-13: 978-0-9818482-0-4

Mommy's Gone to Treatment
Denise D. Crosson, Ph.D., illustrated by Mike Motz • $14.95 US
ISBN-13: 978-0-9799869-1-8

Mommy's Coming Home from Treatment
Denise D. Crosson, Ph.D., illustrated by Mike Motz • $14.95 US
ISBN-13: 978-0-9799869-4-9

JOURNALS

My First Year in Recovery: A Journal for the Journey (Second Edition)
The Editors of Central Recovery Press • $19.95 US
ISBN-13: 978-0-9818482-4-2

My Five-Year Recovery Planner: Looking to the Future,
One Day at a Time
The Editors of Central Recovery Press • $19.95 US
ISBN-13: 978-0-9818482-9-7

My Pain Recovery Journal
The Editors of Central Recovery Press • $17.95 US
ISBN-13: 978-0-9799869-7-0

PAIN RECOVERY

A Day without Pain
Mel Pohl, MD, FASAM • $14.95 US • ISBN-13: 978-0-9799869-5-6

Pain Recovery: How to Find Balance and Reduce Suffering
from Chronic Pain
Mel Pohl, MD, FASAM; Frank J. Szabo, Jr., LADC; Dan Shiode, Ph.D.;
Rob Hunter, Ph.D. • $20.95 US • ISBN-13: 978-0-9799869-9-4

Pain Recovery for Families: How to Find Balance When Someone Else's
Chronic Pain Becomes Your Problem Too
Mel Pohl, MD, FASAM; Frank J. Szabo, Jr., LADC; Dan Shiode, Ph.D.;
Rob Hunter, Ph.D. • $20.95 US • ISBN-13: 978-0-9818482-3-5

Meditations for Pain Recovery
Tony Greco • $16.95 US • ISBN 13: 978-0-9818482-8-0